Musings From MAG...

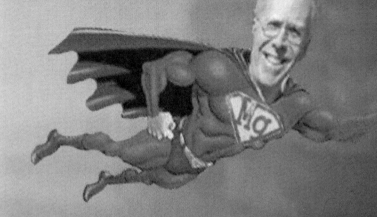

volume three

Compiled By
Genelle Young

**MAGNESIUM
ADVOCACY
GROUP**

First edition, December, 2015

Volume III

Compiled by Genelle Young with permission of Morley Robbins

©2015, Genelle Young and Morley Robbins

Thank you to Michelle Stewart for Editing Support.
Thank you to Megan Young for Cover design, and Editing Support..

Disclaimer:

All information provided here out is completely general, and not specific to any one person. You need to know your mineral status, and have it interpreted by a trained interpreter to know which information would apply to you. Morley is happy to work with you to achieve optimum health via his website, for which a link is provided below. But, I am by no means qualified to do so and do not, at this current time, have the capacity to independently diagnose someone with any mineral deficiency. I am however willing to make suggestions based on my own knowledge.

All recommended supplements and products, at the time of this file being complied, was recommended to Morley and he advises the use of them based on research and information he has come across. He is in no way responsible for any unforeseen side-effects or issue that arise from the direct use of recommended products, nor am I. As companies develop their products, they may be altered in regards to their ingredients, so please check carefully and ask questions in regards to what you intend to take. You need to make sure you are getting what you need and that the supplements you are taking do not counteract each other.

Morley gets no throw back from these products in any way, so his opinion is not governed by any company and what is sold to you does not benefit him in any way. Please be advised that you should not avoid a proper consultation, do not self-diagnose or treat yourself based on the information provided to you, seek a professional opinion.

Morley encourages you to take responsibility for your own health care decisions based upon inspired research, and in partnership with a qualified health care professional who can think well outside the box of today's vogue, misguided, biologically-incorrect, but "politically-correct" medical and dietary recommendations that are fueling the epidemic of chronic disease worldwide.

Hi, my name is Genelle Young.

After following to Magnesium Advocacy Group for some time due to health issues, I decided to take the plunge and do the HTMA with Morley last January. It was such a relief for someone to put on paper that, "yes there is something out of balance". I had seen so many specialists and had so many tests over the years, a Diagnostic Physician even commented "You have been this way so long, so obviously you have learnt to live with it, it's not killing you, and what do you want me to do?"

I had tried endless alternative medicine and to be honest, when I looked into mineral balancing, I was not filled with confidence. And, not to mention, we all know the impact alternative choices can have on the old bank account. While I followed the wall, I would scroll in anticipation for Morley's replied and with great excitement, I would copy his notes. These notes grew and grew and grew. So, it was then that I started thinking that I could share these notes, knowing there had to be other people out there scrolling as I do, waiting for Morley's input, but felt it only right to ask Morley for his blessing. Morley's reply was, "Let's make this an Ebook". I was ecstatic, Morley Robbins wants to work with me?!

And so began the long hours of bringing this all together! I hope it just keeps getting bigger and bigger.

My husband (of 19 years) and I have 4 children, 2 girls, 2 boys, between 18 and 5. We also run our own self built retail business, which we have just expanded, and built a mechanic workshop onto. With so much spare time (can you hear my sarcasm here?), I thought, too easy! Not. (Does anyone else have any idea how much stuff Microsoft Word can do when you actually know how to use it?!) So, for me this has been a labour of love to assemble hoping that I can help people get a better understanding as to what the mineral balancing can do. I hope these notes I have complied, give you a better understanding that, No, you don't have to accept your aliments. Yes, there is help. I have entrusted Morley to Captain our journey's to better health and I have done HTMA's for all of my family, as we all have our quirks that I was looking to iron out. BUT, Mineral Balancing isn't a quick fix. It is a commitment of at least a year or two and most of all, a lifestyle change to maintain. It's not "let's do one HTMA and hope for the best" it is a long term dedication. But, I am sure when you get to the end of this book, you will be looking for that http://gotmag.org/ to get you started too.

I hope you enjoy the information, as much as I did compiling it!!!

Table of Contents

A FEW WORDS ABOUT MAGNESIUM MAN

Morley M. Robbins

"There is no such thing as "medical disease..." There is only "metabolic dysfunction" that is CAUSED by "mineral deficiencies..."

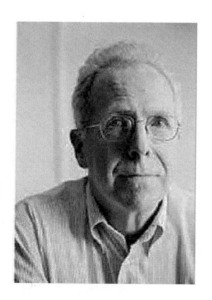

https://www.facebook.com/groups/MagnesiumAdvocacy/

http://gotmag.org/

morley@gotmag.com

847.922.8061

MAGNESIUM ADVOCACY GROUP Founder Morley M. Robbins (aka. "Magnesium Man") has a mainstream medical industry background. That's intriguing when you consider that he is now devoted to promoting natural and preventive health solutions.

Morley had been a hospital executive and consultant for 32 years when, several years ago, he developed a condition called "frozen shoulder." His family doctor quickly recommended surgery as the only hope for Morley if he wanted to be able to lift his right hand above his waist ever again.

Friends who owned a health food store intervened and encouraged Morley to try chiropractic care. His initial response:

"Thanks guys, but I don't do witchcraft."

Several months later, the pain was wearing on him, and his friends insisted.

It only took a couple weeks of "light touch chiropractic care" (Network Spinal Analysis) before his shoulder had full range of motion once again.

The experience was so life-changing for Morley, he questioned everything he knew — or thought he knew — about healing.

He left the world of hospital administration and became a Wellness Coach.

MORLEY DISCOVERS MAG

In July 2011, Morley was guided to read Carolyn Dean's wonderful book *The Magnesium Miracle*. He realized that nutrients, in general and magnesium, in particular, were a key piece of the whole health puzzle that virtually no practitioners seemed to be aware of — even in the natural health world.

He was captivated by this mineral, and went on to read even more. Much more...

Twenty-five books and 2500 articles (and counting) on Mineral metabolism (IE Cp and Iron overload; etc.) Magnesium, Iron and Copper deficiency, Morley has come to realize that Magnesium and key minerals play a role in *all* KEY metabolic systems, and is therefore a contributing factor to nearly *all* major health issues.

Magnesium deficiency is the common thread for millions of Americans who are dealing with **heart disease, diabetes, obesity, osteoporosis, cancer, general fatigue, and any chronic condition borne out of inflammation**.

As Morley read and made connections between hundreds of scientific studies, what he found was shocking:

Magnesium deficiency, or insufficiency, was at the center of all these common modern diseases due to its central role in activating 3,751 proteins, and thus thousands of enzyme systems (far more than the Internet figure of 300 enzyme pathways...).

It became increasingly easy to see why this family of Magnesium-related health problems would be so common in modern life. Over the past century, drinking water treatment and food processing has removed naturally-occurring Magnesium from our dietary environment. Meanwhile stressful lifestyles cause our bodies to burn through what little Magnesium we do have inside us. Furthermore, many prescription medications are known to cause Magnesium, and other mineral loss, as well.

Morley has coined the phrase "Magnesium Burn Rate" (MBR) to help folks internalize the physical price they pay from the many "Stressors!" in their world.

Morley, in concert with his partner, "Dr. Liz" Erkenswick, DC, (who MAG-ically healed his shoulder...) began working with their clients on a program of natural healing, with particular emphasis on this "Magnesium deficiency issue."

Because of Magnesium, their clients' lives changed. Profoundly.

Their clients' "need" for statins, anti-depressants, digestive meds, sleeping pills, and osteoporosis medications (just to name a few) were effectively offset by concerted efforts to manage their stress response, eating REAL foods rich in minerals, vitamins and fats, and undertaking protocols to restore bio-available Magnesium supplements. (3 Steps to Restore Magnesium)

Morley had read the published studies on how Magnesium repletion could help reverse high cholesterol, cure low-grade depression, stop insomnia, increase bone density, and support hundreds of numerous other enzyme-dependent (and thus Magnesium-dependent) processes in the body...

But it was seeing the results in his clients' lives that really galvanized his purpose.

Today, Morley views it as his life's work to push back the tides of nutritional insanity and Magnesium deficiency in the day-to-day lives of inhabitants of Planet Earth!

Through MAG, he is committed to educating as many people as possible about the *MAG-nificence of Magnesium* and ending the epidemic of Magnesium deficiency plaguing the health and well-being of American society. Please join him in his Facebook Magnesium Advocacy Group to gain greater insights into the importance of minerals, in general, and Magnesium, in particular:

https://www.facebook.com/groups/MagnesiumAdvocacy/

TRAINING

Morley did his primary HTMA training with Rick Malter, PhD, www.malterinstitute.org/ Morley has been guided by a dozen other gifted mineral researches and experts, also.

~ A WORD FROM THE MAN HIMSELF ~

It's a bit more complicated than just one program and mentorship, although Rick Malter, PhD has been legendary:

o   I'm a Scorpio -- I LOVE to dig... .

o   I'm a contrarian -- I delight in challenging authority for sport...

o   I'm a conspiracist -- turns out it's NOT a conspiracy...

o   I failed miserably in college to study "science" so I could be a "doctor" -- got "No thanks!" from 18 schools... Ouch! (*And thank God for that!...*)

o   Discovered I had a gift for pattern recognition... Studied General Systems Theory in B-School and loved it!

o   Completed Reed Davis' FDN Program– highly recommend it!

o   Completed 2 of 3 levels of Freddie Ulan, DC's program Nutritional Response Testing -- MIND-BLOWING program...

o   Attended several seminars with Stuart White, DC -- a profoundly gifted practitioner, healer and educator...

o   I was blessed to connect with my now wife, Dr. Liz, who is also a most gifted healer who taught me what natural healing is ALL about -- awakening the innate wisdom of the individual...

o   Read Carolyn Dean, MD, ND's book, "The Magnesium Miracle," that changed my life... (Mostly for the better...)

o   Went on to read 25+ books or more and 2500 articles... And is still digging!...

o   Completed the Institute for Integrated Nutrition program... It's a wonderful program as it exposes you to 50+ different approaches to nutrition... it is, however, a "mineral desert" when it comes to training...

o   I would be remiss to not mention my buddy, Peter Wisniewski (founder of http://endobalance.com/) who was the ONE who actually suggested I get into HTMA analysis and then withstood months (years) of my "bitching" about how hard it was to understand and master... He also has been instrumental in teaching Dr. Liz and me about the amazing gifts of Standard Process supplements, that are magically designed for natural healing...

o   It was because of Pete's suggestion that I took Rick Malter's course which I HIGHLY recommend to anyone seeking to practice HTMA analysis...

I have had the added blessing of forging a friendship since 2009 with Rick that has shaped my thinking as a practitioner, but more importantly, as an awakened participant on this Planet!...

o   And last, but not least, was the two years I spent interacting with Patrick Sullivan Jr. during my time being sponsored by Jigsaw Health (2011-2013). Patrick is simply a class act (by the way, apples don't fall far from trees...) and he "created" the persona of "Magnesium Man!," fostered my confidence as a writer and speaker, and engaged in countless hours of dialogue about how best to communicate the gift of minerals, in general, and Maggie, in particular...

That ^^^^ is the looooong and short of my "training" as it were...

I'm confident that I'll start a "school" but the question is when... Likely in 2016 or 2017. Thank you all for taking an interest...

HI FROM MORLEY

I am most OPEN to learning how to better use these diagnostic tools and welcome the input of other practitioners to learn from. As I've stated repeatedly, I don't pretend to have all the answers -- hardly.

What I do know, however, is that there's a great deal of confusion in conventional circles, in large part due to a failure to understand and incorporate mineral metabolism into the dynamics of metabolic dysfunction...

I have spent 32+ years as an executive in the health care field... I made a very conscious choice in 2009, to step off the Allopathic grid and enlighten souls about how their bodies REALLY work, not how BIG Pharma and their Minion Deities want them to believe it works...

Please know, I don't pretend to have all the answers... Truly I don't. I do however, have a very different perspective on human metabolism, based on the mineral foundation that run the body.

What I can say is that I have NO fear of standing with an umbrella in the face of a TIDAL WAVE of "D"isinformation and "D"eception that floods MOST conventinal articles and research on health, nutrition and healing.

We have been Misled... We have been Misfed... Truth be known, we have Missing Minerals -- mostly!

I have "recognised" degrees:

O   "PhD", which stands for "Passionate hatred for Disinformation"... And an o   "MD", which stands for "Mineral Detective."

Each of which are "Honorary" and bestowed to me by the Wizard of Oz!

MAG is littered with hundreds (thousands?...) of folks who have been abused by an insensitive, arrogant, and in my humble opinion, under trained medical system devoid of common sense or willingness to sort out the metabolic foundation revealed by minerals...

There are hundreds of folks who requested the Mag RBC only to get a serum Mg which is entirely worthless as a diagnostic tool. Yet doctors continually order serum Mg. largely due to their limited training.

As for the cost, it can be expensive, but there, too, many, many folks have WASTED thousands of $$£££€€¥¥ in the vortex of conventional medicine...

Trust me, I hear upward of twenty five stories per week -- each one more heart-breaking than the last... The level of clinical incompetence is mind-numbing, quite frankly.

So, my sincere recommendation to ALL, is to take action -- outside the BOX of convention -- and take control of your health and steps to bring your body back into balance.

And in closing, I would encourage all to STOP "hoping and praying" that your doctor will finally figure this out. Their training is designed to treat disease - NOT cure it. There are many theories on "why" this is the case. All are speculative. The bottom lome is they are NOT trained in minerals... PERIOD!!

Of the 33,000 MAG-pies, I know of only 3 MDs who have publicly declared their training...

Converntinal practitioners are not exactly flocking to my Facebook page -- nor am I expecting them to -- and **nor should you, either**...

I am growing weary of "labels" that the average person fears and the average practitioner does NOT fully understand, metabolically.

100% of the people on the MAG group are "Stress! Cadets" and thus mineral deserts... from 3-4 generations of overly processed foods, as well as abject denial re the vital importance of minerals to run the body

Welcome to new MAG members.

Here's the link to Mildred S. Seelig, MD, MPH Magnus Opus: re the fundemental ESSENTIALITY of Mg in our lives.

http://www.mgwater.com/.../Magnesium.../preface.shtml

That will keep you occupied for a couple of weeks, at least...

And please know we've never met a question we didn't enjoy!

AFFILIATED PRACTITIONERS

HTMA Practitioners affiliated with the Magnesium Advocacy Group

Morley Robbins, CHC

Rick Malter, PhD

Robert Thompson, MD

Julie Casper, LAc

Pippa Galea

Wendy Myers

Eileen Durphy

Dede Moore – EFT Practitioner

EFT aka Emotional Freedom Technique is "acupuncture without the needles", with an added emotional component. We cannot separate body from mind. This is an easy and amazing tool to boost and promote your overall heath, as well as eradicate issues that you think are only physical.

A couple of reasons to use EFT:

1) It is an easy and effective way to handle stress and reduce our MBR.

2) If you have tried several things to physically feel better, and they're not working.

3) You consider your past or your present full of "Stressful!" or emotional situations.

4) People drawn to this issue of minerals and mineral deficiency tend to be smart people. Smart people like to be optimal. For EFT to work its MAG-ic, we need to "surrender" to the process. That is BEST done with a trained practitioner.

A couple of reasons to work with a certified EFT Practitioner:

1) They are trained to see what you can't see. For example, you might think you need to work on your marriage when really there is an issue from your childhood.

2) In EFT lingo you are borrowing the benefits which means you actually benefit from the energy of the trained Practitioner.

3) If you want to get to the Olympics competing as a runner you wouldn't just run on your own, you would get a trainer.

Members of the MAG group are fortunate enough to have a very gifted EFT Practitioner among us! Dede Moore generously offers the first session free. You can contact Dede at eft4anxiety@gmail.com

I took Dede up on her standing offer to the MAG-pie community: One free EFT session to try it. I have been doing weekly sessions for the past 4-5 months and was blown away by what it has done for me. Dede is incredibly gifted in her skills, she has applied this AMAZING EFT tool to a number of key issues, (aka, emotional knots) and they are GONE!...

I am very grateful that our paths crossed and that she is so talented at what she does. I would encourage you and any others, who are dealing with emotional issues at the core of their mineral imbalances – which would be 100% of us!!! Again, emotional "stressors!" Is often the origin of the Mg Burn Rate.

MINERALS

Magnesium: A Beginners Guide To Mag

Even though roughly over 80+% of the population is Mg deficient, we still recommend testing first.

http://gotmag.org/magnesium-deficiency-101/

o   Mg RBC (functional range is 6.0-7.0mg/dL, strive for 6.5)

http://requestatest.com/magnesium-rbc-testing

o   Hair Tissue Mineral Analysis

http://gotmag.org/work-with-us/

o   How to Restore Mg:

http://gotmag.org/how-to-restore-magnesium/

o   Critical co-fractor for Mg absorption:

-      B6 helps get Magnesium INSIDE the cell (recommended brands are Jigsaw Health mg SRT and Magkey as they contain B6, Mg co-factor.)

-      Boron helps KEEP mag INSIDE the cell (Anderson's Concentrated Minerals or Aussie Sea Minerals, Relyte, as well are prunes and raisins, contain the much needed trace mineral, boron.)

- Sodium Bicarbonate helps get Mag Inside the Mitochondria. (Mag water)

- Selenium and Taurine and are added co-factors to improve Mg intake and retention...

Where Mg is found in our body:

SAVINGS: 60% in bones. (Bone matrix)

CHECKING: 27% in muscles with the highest concentration in the ventricles of the heart.

DEBIT: 17% in soft tissue (heart, brain, liver, kidney, endocrine glands and related tissue.

WALLET: 1% in the blood it comes out of "storage" in tissue and components of the blood 1st, bones 2nd, and lastly from serum which is why Mg serum tests are worthless.

MAGNESIUM: HOW TO RESTORE MAG

I am often asked, "So how much Magnesium do I need to take daily?"

It's a great question. And like most great questions, the answer is, "It depends."

There are actually 3 points to consider:

1) Increased S*T*R*E*S*S = Increased MBR

First, please know that stress consumes Magnesium (Mg) — it's how we're wired as a species. **The more "Stress!" you are under, the more Magnesium your body burns.**

I call this the "Magnesium Burn Rate", or MBR. It's the metabolic price we pay for all that pressure, tension and change we all feel.

Take an inventory of the dimensions of stress... Food allergies, dependence on processed food, exposure to heavy metals, use of Rx drugs, and the granddaddy of them all — mental and emotional stress, to name but a few of the "Stressors" that deplete our Mg stores. Take whatever steps you can to mitigate these issues to shore up these Mg leaks.

And when you know your "Stress!"/MBR is increasing, know that your body will be craving more Magnesium.

2) What is your Current Magnesium Status?

The most efficient and cost-effective way to get a reading on your current Magnesium status is to order the MagRBC blood test (available from Request a Test).

This simple test costs $49 and you'll usually have results emailed to you within 72 hours, for those that resides within the states.

The current Lab reference range is 4.2 – 6.8 mg/dL, but know that in 1962 (before every 1/3 person was obese, diabetic or addicted to Rx meds) the Reference Range was 5.0-7.0mg/dL (** / 2.43 for mmol/L). Based on this latter Range, any score below 6.0 mg/dL is a clear signal of Magnesium deficiency. Ideally, we **STRIVE** to get the Mag RBC to **6.5**, 7 is Heaven!

If you have many Magnesium deficiency symptoms (http://gotmag.org/magnesium-deficiency-101/), an even less expensive option is to just start increasing your Magnesium intake. See the next step…

3) Protocol for Restoring Magnesium

- **Diet** – Start eating more Magnesium-rich foods: Seafood, especially kelp and oysters. Whole grains, especially buckwheat, millet and wild rice. Leafy greens, especially Collards, Beet Greens, Mustard Greens, spinach and kale. Nuts and seeds, especially cashews, almonds, and pistachio nuts, as well as pumpkin seeds.

And everyone's favorite, Chocolate! But, only dark chocolate with a high content of Cacao, 80% or more is best!

(NOTE: Because of mineral depletion in the soil and modern food processing methods, I've determined that it's basically impossible to get enough Magnesium from food alone, so please continue reading…)

- **Magnesium Mineral Drops** – Put Anderson's Concentrated Mineral, or Aussie Sea Minerals or Relyte, drops in your water — minerals are the *other* "element" we're looking for when we're thirsty for H2O!

- **Magnesium Oil Footbath's** – Do a magnesium oil footbath. If you can't do it daily, at least 2-3X/week to replenish extreme magnesium deficiency rapidly.

Dose is 1 - 2 oz of Magnesium Oil plus ½ cup of Baking Soda + ½ Tbsp Borax in enough hot water to cover your toes in a small tub.

- **Epsom Salt/Mg Chloride Flakes Bath** – Magnesium baths are great. Grandma used to recommend them for just about everything! And Epsom Salt (Magnesium Sulfate) is readily available at just about every local drugstore, and Mg Cl flakes at your local health food store.

Dose is 1-2 cups of Epsom Salt OR Mg Cl flakes (NEVER TOGETHER) + 1 Cup of Baking Soda (*not* baking powder) + 1 Tbsp Borax, and immerse yourself in this rejuvenating liquid for 30-40 min. I recommend slowing down and enjoying one per week.

Please know Mg Chloride oil out performs Epsom Salt if the objective is to increase Mg levels... Epsom salt, however, is superior for detox... I've studied this carefully with clients and those with the fastest rise in Mg status all make liberal use of Mg Chloride oil, either through baths or transdermal spray...

But if "slowing down" isn't in your vocabulary, continue reading...

- **Magnesium Supplements** – Take a bio-available Magnesium supplement *every* day.

Three brands that I confidently recommend are Jigsaw Magnesium with SRT (time release), Magnesium Glycinate by Pure Encapsulations, and MagKey.

(NOTE: No matter what magnesium supplement you use, be sure to also supplement with vitamin B6, an important co-factor to Magnesium absorption. To this point, I give a slight edge to Jigsaw and MagKey since their formulas already include B6.)

The Recommended Daily Intake (RDI) of Magnesium is 400 mg. But I believe the Optimal Daily Dose is 650 mg for Women and 850 mg for men, but please vary it based upon your daily Magnesium Burn Rate.

My preferred rule of thumb is to take 5 mg/lb or 10 mg/kg your body weight in mg's of Mg (e.g. If you weigh 100 lbs or 50 kg, take 500 mg's Mg.) That is to maintain your Mg status, take more to restore, or address your increased MBR.

Again, the focus here is on "optimum" dosing, not daily "minimum" intakes.

4) One Last Thing…

OK, now this last part is quite difficult, so please pay close attention… I'd like you to do this degree of Mg supplementation each and every day. We have THREE key daily absolutes: Air, Water, Magnesium — YES, it's that important!

And when you start increasing your Magnesium intake, you'll be fueling your body with *the* Master Mineral that powers *all* 100 Trillion cells, especially the largest muscle in your body, your non-stop beating heart.

MAGNESIUM: WHAT'S YOUR MAG STATUS

Please know that the MAG functional Range for optimal Health is 5.0-7.0mg/dL. 6.5 is optimal, 7 is heaven. [**mg/dl /2.43mmol/L**] (PLease know, the current lab range is based on very chronically ill people...)

When Mg is deficient, here's what's impacted:

o   Autonomic Nervous System gets agitated

o   Energy Production (ATP production) our response to "Stress!" gets aggrivated.

o   3,751 proteins are affected, especailly those in the mitochondria.

o   Iron absorption and transport is affected which lead to Anemia...

o   B12 can't get INSIDE the cell (the enzyme is dependent on Mg-ATP!), and builds up in the blood...

Suggestion, do your best to bypass the Xanax as it will only further deplete your Mg, Cu, Zn and Fe, work on restoring your Mg status
www.gotmag.org/how-to-restore-magnesium/

Pursue multiple channels of Mg recovery... BEFORE you resort to shots, etc.

MAGNESIUM: DEFICIENCY SYMPTOMS

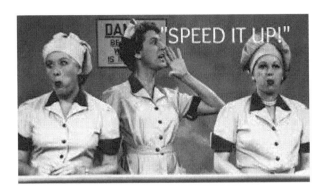

What causes MAG loss....

Physical, Metabolic, Emotional, Environmental, Electrical and Nutritional "Stress!"

Among the MOST damaging sources of Mg Loss:

o   Exposure to Fluoride...
o   Anesthesia...
o   Rx medications...
o   Emotional Shock (death of a loved one, etc.)
o   Car Accidents.
o   Iron overload.

These are some good sources for you...

http://bja.oxfordjournals.org/content/83/2/302.full.pdf

http://ckj.oxfordjournals.org/content/5/Suppl_1.toc

http://www.mgwater.com/Seelig/Magnesium-Deficiency-in-the-Pathogenesis-of-Disease/preface.shtml

http://www.lifeextension.com/magazine/2008/5/Magnesium-Widespread-Deficiency-With-Deadly-Consequences/Page-01

http://www.mgwater.com/rodtitle.shtml

That ought to keep you in the Library for at least a couple of hours...

There's plenty more where those came from...

As a former "hospital jockey," I had NO idea how CENTRAL Magnesium was to optimal health or how its deficiency was the CAUSE to most, if not ALL, chronic disease.

Picture a "hub and spoke" wheel. At the core is Mg deficiency, and the spokes are the hundreds/thousands of enzyme pathways --that are Mag dependent-- that when they stop firing, CAUSE the conditions that we have been "trained" to believe is "disease." They are NOT disease. They are nutritional deficiencies, that manifest as symptoms and pain...

Even "auto-immune" conditions...

http://www.rense.com/general83/fount.htm

http://www.nutritionalmagnesium.org/magnesium-deficiency-in-autoimmune-disease/

The resilience of the human body exceeds anything I know of... Remove the "Stressors!" and feed the body balanced nutrients, and my reading of the literature suggests that virtually all conditions are reversible...

For those that will come down hard on me for saying that, it just may be that we have NOT learned how to do the above in all its forms...

Part of the challenge in our health recovery, is our limited belief in the "lack of reversibility..." Or the "lack of resilience" of the human metabolism.

MAGNESIUM: MAG YOUR BATH

Epsom Salt is more of a detox...

Mg Chloride flakes is more of a source for Mg restoration...

Mg Cl flakes are uses to make Mg Cl oil or to place in a tub for a bath... it's more long-term recovery...

Epsom salts (Mg SO4) is another form of Mg that is used for bathing... its more short-term relief

Baking Soda (Sodium Bicarbonate) is added to water to make it more Alkaline... It does NOT contain Borax... You can use up to 2 Cup/bath...

Borax (Boron) is a mineral with known properties to help regulate the Calcium/Magnesium dance... Yes the washing power!!! 1 Tbsp is a good dose for each full bath, or 1/2 Tbsp for each foot bath.

MAGNESIUM: MILK OF MAGNESIA MOM

MoM was invented in 1873 and has been used throughout the world for ~150 years... It has KNOWN properties as BOTH an antiacid and a laxative. Why is it being banned in Europe, U.K. and Down Under?!?

BECAUSE IT WORKS!!!

All is NOT as it seems...

Please read this slooooowly:

http://monthlyaspectarian.com/morley-August-2012.html

I can properly speak far more eloquently to the efforts underway around the Globe to restrict access to minerals and supplements to non-Priestly group of citizens that make up the 99.9% of the population.

It is a dark, dark chapter in the evolution of the world...

That said, I have NO insider information on why this is happening. What I have noted is that the following Mg-based products are more, and more impossible to find:

o   Carter's Liver pills...
o   Doan's Back pills...
o   Bufferin (Aspirin buffered with Mg!)
o   and numerous others...

And what are these being replaced with? NSAIDS!

And what's a distinctive feature of NSAIDs?

They create Magnesium loss...

Hmmmmm... Think that's a coincidence?... Nope, me neither!

Please note Bullet #3 in the attached article:
http://www.askdrmaxwell.com/2012/10/do-you-have-a-magnesium-deficiency/

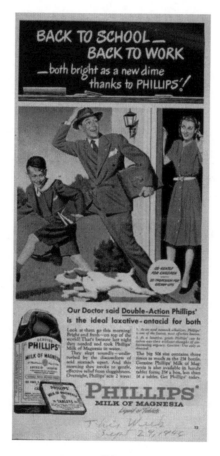

MOTHER WAS RIGHT: THE HEALTH BENEFITS OF MILK OF MAGNESIA

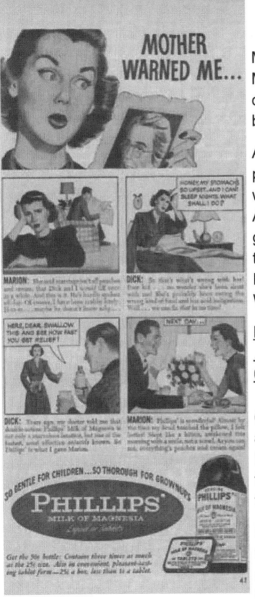

MAG-pies of the "Mother" Persuasion -- Alert!

May one and ALL of the Moms that grace this MOM-crazed group have a blessed and wonderful Day!

And as a MAG-appropriate present, I present to you the wonderful writing of Marshall Alan Wolf, MD, one of the greatest Cardiologists to train future such doctors at Harvard's Brigham and Women's Hospital...

http://www.ncbi.nlm.nih.gov/.../PMC150.../pdf/tacca117000001.pdf

(I was absolutely humbled and honoured to chat with him a couple of years ago to thank him for and to discuss this delightful article...)

May you find comfort and wisdom in his observations about BOTH his Mom, and Maggie!...

MAGNESIUM: MORLEY'S MAG OBSESSION

Is it "healthy" to be obsessed with magnesium?

As a nation, we've been "taught" to be obsessed with:

o   Calcium...
o   Cholesterol...
o   "Low Fat!"...
o   Tons of "D!"...
o   No Salt!...
o   No Red Meat...
o   No Eggs!...
o   and on, and on, and on, and on...

All of which has been proven to be pure poppycock! (Yes, even the vaulted "D"ietary "D"ictum on "D" is "D"ying... Thank God!)

At least by focusing on Maggie, we're restoring the metabolic foundation of the human body to resume its natural role in quietly regulating and balancing and energizing thousands upon thousands of functions that allow us to be symptom-free and Rx med-free!

In my humble opinion, it beats our earlier programming by factors thousands-fold...Truly, why are people wasting their time trying to "convince" their doctor regarding a Mg blood test?!?

What was most telling in that exchange: "If Mg were important they would test for it."

The FACT that the doctor does NOT test for it SAYS IT ALL FOLKS!...

It's not just "important," it's CENTRAL to understanding the metabolic health of the individual, and the fact that you've never heard that before does NOT mean it is wrong...

Sheeeeseeesh...

When was the last time you updated your understanding of the extensive network of metabolic, detox and energy pathways that are ENTIRELY dependent on Mg status?...

There are countless secondary and tertiary pathways that begin to malfunction when the cell, and key enzyme pathways, are no longer able to produce energy (Mg-ATP) efficiently...

If you are relying on the filtered textbook(s) of Physiology that you studied in Medical School, your knowledge base is seriously flawed... more like "Swiss Cheese," than based on definitive science...

I don't take lightly to "practitioners" who received their education from BIG Pharma-funded schools of Rx dispensing acting as "experts" on "disease" when they have flawed education...

Be ready for significant and scientific pushback on my end with a clear intent of informing the masses that when ALL THE DUST settles, the ultimate hinge for disease and dysfunction is a LACK OF ENERGY" (Mg-ATP) that is largely a Mg status issue -- induced by a wide spectrum of "Stressors!" just as Karl Fiedler, MD, theorized in 1899, and his protégé, Hans Selye, MD, PhD, ScD was able to prove in the 30,000 experiments that he conducted with all manner of species during his illustrious and storied 50-yr career defining and codifying the General Adaptation Syndrom (GAS) tha is the intellectial bedrck of "Stress!" And its impact on our physicology adn immune system...

MAGNESIUM: REACTIONS

There are ~25 different forms of Maggie... I know not why, but we all do not respond well to different forms...

Hang in there and see how you respond to other forms...

In chatting with a noted pathologist about the "accuracy" of the Mag RBC test, he pointed out that the error can be up to +/- 20%, which is a significant # when you think about it...

Point.... Counter Point...

o   Mg Malate and Mg Glycinate are among the MOST effective in their absorption and impact... These are our "go to" oral Mg supplements...

o   Mg Cl oil -- transdermal -- has been used successfully for thousands of generations by folks who live near the Sea...

o   Mg Taurate is a wonderful form that is especially effective for those dealing with Heart muscle issues...

o   Mg Citrate is well absorbed, but MANY are affected by the fact that the Citrate molecule irritates the intestinal lining... Moving waste via "irritation" is NOT the same as metabolic "stimulation..."

o   Epsom salt (Mg Sulfate) has been used effectively since the LATE 1500's as a powerful detox and relaxing agent...

o   Mg Hydroxide (MoM) is MOST effective -- when used properly. Its use and effectiveness since its discovery in the late 1800's is legendary... MJ Hamp has a proven use for making Mg water that has helped MANY MAG-Pies on this FB Group...

o   Mg Threonate is the latest, but is NOT the only Mg to cross the BBB. It IS the form that has the BEST PR campaign that is designed to convince you that "Patented" Minerals is the way to go! (You should be VERY worried about THAT aspect of this product...)

Albion Minerals is the source for Jigsaw's Mg SRT and the two forms of Mg Glycinate that we use in our wellness center in Louisiana: Doctor's Best, and PURE Encapsulations...

Keep in mind, Jigsaw INCLUDES the needed B's (And YES, the Folate is the RIGHT kind...) and the Mg Glycinate requires the addition of the B6, etc.

Magnesium's role in the body is to regulate levels of thousands of of proteins that then affect minerals, vitamins, enzymes, hormones, neurotransmitters, and genes...

Maggie is powerful mineral that plays a key role in many, many, many activities.

It's important to know that Cortisol is your friend and when it's low, it's likely that you've got too little Potassium, brought on by Adrenal Fatigue that becomes Adrenal Suppression that causes a systemic loss of Sodium and Potassium. And excess Calcium, bio-unavailable Copper and Hormone-D work wonders to keep the Potassium in a state of deficiency...

It's a very dynamic process, and while hard to believe, is kept in balance and in motion when the body is allowed to keep its Magnesium status at optimal levels... It truly is the "Conductor of the Cell's Orchestra of Minerals..."

If you get lighted headed when starting Mag:

o   It's important to understand that the Adrenals are RULED
        by the mineral ratio of Sodium/Magnesium (Na/Mg)

o   Very likely, your Adrenals are whipped, which means that
        your Sodium (Na) is on the LOW side...

o   The infusion of Mg causes the Na/Mg ratio to get more
        inverted, thus slooooowing you down more.

o   Very likely, you need Adrenal support to elevate your
        Sodium as the "light headed" feeling is associated with
        low Sodium which then affects fluid volume...

I would advise three things:

1)   Get a broad based assessment of your minerals, via an
        HTMA

2)   Read and act on this:
        http://gotmag.org/how-to-restore-magnesium/

3)   Take the Adrenal Cocktail to support your body's need for
        minerals to feed the Adrenals...

Knowing you're "whipped," that's what I'd do... take several days
(up to 2 weeks) to nourish the Adrenals with the minerals they've
been missing and then start up the Maggie, again, but do so
slooooooowly...

Getting tired following an infusion of Maggie is either a possible
Detox reaction (pathways get fired up when Mg-ATP is around...)
or it is a sign of weak Adrenals, given that these "Stress!" Glands
are ruled by the mineral ratio of Sodium/Mg. So, when you pump

in a lot of Mg, without mineral and vitamin support for the Adrenals, the ratio goes south and so, too, does your energy level.

The unintended backside to "Mo' Maggie" is that it can cause an inversion in the Adrenal Ratio (Na/Mg). The BIGGER the Mg, the more it can drive the Adrenal Ratio South which will cause you to feel "exhausted!" I wonder if that might not be part of your dynamic...

You might want to try Adrenal Cocktail and see how you respond to some targeted Adrenal support...

One way you can test whether this latter issue is the cause is to try the Adrenal Cocktail 2-3 times and see how your respond to an infusion of targeted minerals (Sea Salt and Potassium [Cream of Tartar])

1/4 tsp Sea Salt
1/4 tsp Cream of Tartar (Potassium)
1/2 cup of Fresh squeezed Orange or Lime Juice (NOT Store bought!...)

Drink at 10am and/or 3pm and see how you feel for several days...

80% of folks who try this feel energized, the other 20% -- not so much. And thats ok, there are other options, but this is the easiest and most fundamental approach.

Ultimately, you'll need focused nutritional support for your Adrenals, assuming that this is a key factor (which I suspect it is...), but this will give you support in the interim...

Just like adding oil to your car engine, it's always best to check the "dipstick" to find out how low you REALLY are... and this is true of people and minerals, too...

Best way to assess this is via an HTMA... This is discussed here:

www.gotmag.org/work-with-us/

Totally agree that "Adrenal Support" is needed in addition to the Adrenal Cocktail. At the end of the day, these "Stress!" Glands need to be re-built and re-energise... which is accelerated with the use of herbal adaptogens, like Ashwaganda, Rhodiola, Licorice Root, holy basil etc...

These approaches are very potent and need to be administered with direction of a practitioner, and a proper context that comes from mineral testing (HTMA, etc.) Mg causes **most** to relax, but excites some... I wish I knew why...

The reasons for "agitated" sleep are likely:

o   Excess Calcium (It is the mineral that keeps you in Sympathetic Dominance... "Fight or Flight"...)

o   Excess, unbound Copper and Iron (keeps you in HYPER-Sympathetic Dominance! And they disrupts the Melatonin Pathway -- badly!)

o   Too little Sodium (Electrolyte Derangement is very disruptive...)

o   Too little Potassium (it is the mineral that enables the Parasympathetic response... "Rest and Recovery"...

What keeps these three issues in proper alignment? Optimal Mg status, but without knowing your "mineral wiring" you will be engaged in the "Bill Murray 'Caddyshack' Strategy of Supplementation..."

A foundational starting point is testing and assessing your mineral profile -- not just blindly throwing the latest vitamin or neurotransmitter -- both of which serve at the pleasure of the minerals...

You can be "neurologically switched," which is not uncommon these days with the food additives and environmental toxins. Don't mean to play a wild card here, but folks who have a "HYPER" response to Maggie, need to be sensitive to taking it in the am and may need to assess what other factors may be at play, in this ATYPICAL response.

Please know that each member of the MAG Community has a different biochemical make-up. The fact that one person has a reaction, means that that person has had a reaction and should NOT become a basis of decision-making on your part.

The key here is to understand that Mineral restoration, with a particular emphasis on Maggie, is the key strategy for our metabolic function and dis-ease elimination. What is important is for you to experiment with different forms of Mg and determine what works in YOUR body...

Again, this is explained here:

www.gotmag.org/how-to-restore-magnesium/

Please take the time to engage in testing to have a proper

mineral context for the efforts that you'll undertake with your diet and nutrition...

It is a very rare thing for Americans to be able to eat enough Magnesium in the typical, processed American diet.

Rare?...

It's more like, "next to impossible!"

Why's that?

o   Fluoride everywhere...

o   Excess dietary and supplement of Calcium and Iron...

o   Excess Hormone-D-- that is "Calcium on Steroids!"

o   Commercial agriculture that is an abomination to food, due to fertilizers, herbicides, etc...

o   Toxic industrial oils, soybean, canola, corn oil, etc...

o   Excess dependence on Magnesuric Rx meds, they casue Mag to exit via the urine...

o   Excess Sugars and HFCS...

o   Excess MSG, burns up minerals...

o   Relentless "Stressors!" that constantly deplete minerals...

And this is just the headlines...

I know that you know this... this is just a reinforces for the MAG-pies!

And, remember those Co-Factors---

These "status quo" RBC results are confounding... Me thinks it is multiple factors that need to be accounted for and addressed:

What is the status of:

o   Plasma Zinc

o   Serum Copper

o   B6 intake

o   Boron

o   Bicarbonate

o   Taurate status (that affects B6)

o   Excess unbound Copper status (that kills Mg, B6 and Zinc!)

o   Excess unbound Iron, that kills Mg, B6 and Zinc!

o   Selenium status, needed for glutathione

o   pH of the body, which is notably affected by "Stressors!"

o   Effect of "Stressors!" not accounted for... [i.e. Mg Blocking Factors (Rx meds, excess Calcium, excess sugars, excess Hormone-D, etc.]

It's unusual to be taking this much Mg and feel no benefit. It suggests the Mg is NOT getting inside the cell.

o   B6 helps get Mg into cell

o   Boron helps keep it in the cell

o   Copper, and Iron has a decided effect on Zinc, B6, and Mg. If the Iron or Copper level are out of control, it is likely the Mg uptake will be challenged. Happy to discuss this further as you have the time and/or interest...

This process of restoring Mg status is VERY MUCH a Debits and Credits phenomenon... It is NOT just about taking Mo' Maggie! It IS about managing the MBR (Mg Burn Rate)... And making sure we are accounting for the Mg leaks as well as the Mg intake -- properly supported with co-factors to get and keep the Mg INSIDE the cells...

"Are you feeling better and are your symptoms melting away?!?." Not an insignificant component that deserves serious consideration...

At the end of the day, I want the MAG-pies to know that the forms of Mg therapy are rich and diverse...

There are compelling success stories whether we are talking about Mg MSM, Chelated Mg, Epsom Salts, Mg drops for water, Mg Bicarbonate, Mg-rich foods...

At first, it will appear a bit overwhelming... but as you become better versed in the MAG-ic of Magnesium, you will find that there are forms that you respond best to. And ideally, you will find 2-3 different forms so as to provide a bit of diversity for your bored little body that has been deprived of this mineral for faaaaar too long.

Don't hesitate to ask questions -- it's why we're here. We want a significant portion of the Planet to discover the role that this foundational mineral plays and that there are numerous ways to bring maggie back to our cells. All forms are welcomed!

Two industries were born from global Magnesium deficiency:

o   Allopathic pharmaceutical industry...(which is largely composed of synthetic chemicals doing the job of Magnesium when it is insufficient inside the human body...)

o   Alternative supplement industry... (Which is largely composed of synthetic-derived supplements made by the very same companies in the 1st bullet point...)

Glycinate can be overstimulating...

I would first encourage you to get a Mag RBC to understand the metabolic origin of your symptoms and the feeling of "Stress!".

Other options: Mg Cl Oil, Mg Water, and/or Mg Malate (Jigsaw), Mg Taurate, or Mg Orotate are proven to absorb well. Mg L-Threonate is another viable option.

o   Please note the Nutrition Therapy of this overview of (MVP) Mitral Valve Prolapse by Dr. Hoffman:

http://drhoffman.com/article/mitral-valve-prolapse-3/

MAGNESIUM: AFFECT ON MANGANESE

I've heard that Mg can affect Mn for years... I've read my fair share of articles on both, but have a decided favorite, as you know...

Can you offer up an article or two that clearly lays out this dynamic?...

I agree with you that many do have a Copper, Iron and Mn deficits -- which CLEARLY show up on HTMAs and are further amplified in blood testing, but their "deficiency" origin is different for each one:

o   Copper -- lack of Ceruloplasmin (Cp) being produced in the Liver...

o   Iron -- lack of bioavailable Copper to fire up the Iron proteins that are ALL Copper dependent... again, due to a lack of Cp...

o   Manganese -- It, too, has a connection with Ceruloplasmin... And of course it's another key divalent cation along with Maggie... I've NEVER read any caution by the hundreds of Mg researchers that I've studied that EVER said, "Now be careful of its impact on Mn..."

But please, set the record straight... And if I'm wrong, I'll apologize and set out to make sure that we clarify this across a lot of FB Groups...

One of the MOST important functions for Mn is to fire up the Mitochondrial Mn-SOD enzyme to neutralize Oxidative Stress that evolves in the process of making ATP...

This is a KEY intracellular function and enzyme. Getting a serum measurement that is HIGH Mn means that this mineral is LEAVING the cell -- I know not why... too much Iron possibly?...

What I neglected to point out is that when Iron shows up LOW, what it's REALLY telling us is that it's being STORED in the Liver, Kidney, Brain, Joints, etc...

It's BEYOND confusing and counter-intuitive, but that's how our bodies work and reveal their dysfunction in these blood tests...

I would strongly encourage a full panel of intracellular minerals that Doctor's Data offers to assess his intracellular mineral/enzyme status...

Given my "Mineral Detective" work, that's where I'd begin...

Manganese and molybdenum helps with the process of sulfur. You can get both from organic brown rice.

Be sure to pre-soak 24 hours before cooking if you go with the rice. Also take vitamin B1 with MSM. Remember MSM helps you to produce your own B vitamins in your body so be aware of cutting back that usage.

MSM also opens up your cells so you may even need to decrease dosages of other RX and minerals.

MAGNESIUM: FACTORS TO CONSIDER

This is one of the better all-round articles on Mg:

http://bja.oxfordjournals.org/content/83/2/302.full.pdf

This is an ENTIRE Journal DEVOTED to this topic. If you take the time to read it, you will be transfixed...

Little chance that that will happen as Mg is treated as a "hood ornament" on a car and NOT the keys to make it work...

http://ckj.oxfordjournals.org/content/5/Suppl_1.toc

http://ckj.oxfordjournals.org/content/5/Suppl_1/i3.full

And let's not forget this BLOCKBUSTER that profiles the fact that 3,751 proteins (enzymes) do NOT work in the human body when Mg is missing...

http://www.ncbi.nlm.nih.gov/pmc/articles/PMC3439678/

Please note, that ALL these articles ^^^ are written OUTSIDE the United States... that is NOT an accident.

Magnesium activates 3,751 proteins (enzymes) in the human body...

There is NO other mineral that even comes close to that impact... (Copper weighs in at ~300, Zinc at ~200...)

When studied at an Oklahoma Medical Center, 92% of doctors NEVER tested for Mg status, and those that did, tested for serum Mg, which in my humble opinion, is a waste of time, €£¥$, and blood...

Ask a Surgeon, how often he tested patients for Mg status, or ensured that Mg was administered during surgery during his/her years as a Surgeon, even though the "Stress!" of surgery and the Fluoride-activated anesthesia DEPLETED Mg in every patient he/she operated on...

And given that EVERY cell of our body runs on ATP, but it doesn't work inside our body unless it's COMPLEXED with Mg, it makes no sense, to me that doctors NEVER test for it... (I guess I'm just goofy that way...)

Thus, the ONLY way to explain this mineral insanity is that it is entirely by design. A scientist would fixate on the mineral that ENSURES energy (I.e. Mg-ATP...) and thousands of enzyme transactions to ensure optimal health. As I see it, doctors are NOT scientists, given their focus on Rx drugs, and NOT minerals that activates enzymes that ensure metabolic homeostasis....

And that is just one Mg Man's opinion...

Please know, the serum measure for Magnesium is a waste of time, blood and $$$... Really!

This is a mineral that RESIDES INSIDE the cell. Serum is a form of blood that resides OUTSIDE the cell. It makes NO sense to use serum Mg as the dipstick. When we are baking cookies, are we fixated on the kitchen room temperature OR oven temperature?

I would advise you to get a Magnesium RBC ASAP. But then we've got to assess your overall mineral status (best done via an HTMA) and then I would advocate a targeted blood test to assess what is causing your perpetual Mg loss, more likely excess, unmanaged Iron.

My hypothesis is that if you have increased Oxidative Stress, it's very likely being triggered by an imbalance of your Zn<>Cu<>Fe dynamic. The blood test that I would recommend is:

http://requestatest.com/mag-zinc-copper-panel-with-iron-panel-testing

Hope that offers some much needed direction. The fact that a doctor is oblivious to this FOUNDATIONAL mechanism of the body should send a decided *chill* down your spine. Note, there is a reason why I refer to these practitioners as "Mineral Denialists."

That designation is both an observation and a condemnation -- they should be mortified by what they DON'T know about the metabolic machinery of the human body, especially Magnesium and the 3,751 proteins that do NOT work when Mg is not at an optimal level...

When we're baking cookies, we're NOT at all concerned about Kitchen (serum Mg) temperature as it doesn't affect the cookies whether it's 68 or 72 degrees in the room.

What we ARE concerned with is whether the Oven (Mag RBC) is at 350 degrees.

Here's the "clinical" answer...

Blood is a transport medium.

It has a VERY TIGHT pH tolerance of 7.35-7.45.

What GUARANTEES that pH is the balance of Electrolytes...

They are managing pH in that medium and have limited metabolic purpose...

The action is INSIDE the cells...

Magnesium (and Potassium) is an Intracellular mineral...

Magnesium works its MAG-ic INSIDE the cells...

It makes NO SENSE to measure an intracellular mineral (Mg) in an extracellular medium (Serum)...

Same explanation without the Chocolate Chips!...

A little "light" reading prior to your next doctor visits...

http://ckj.oxfordjournals.org/content/5/Suppl_1/i15.full

The enzyme that allows Insulin INSIDE the cell is called Tyrosine Kinase... It is Mg-dependent...

(As are 149 of the 150 Kinase enzymes that RUN our cellular machinery...)

The OTHER notable side to the Insulin's NOT working story is that excess, unmanaged Iron in the Pancreas is the metabolic ORIGIN of a lack of Insulin production. Turns out that Beta cells have a wicked attraction to Iron and if Ceruloplasmin is low, as it is in most MAG-Pies, then the excess Iron burns out the pancreas...

MAGNESIUM: CITRATE

http://www.ncbi.nlm.nih.gov/m/pubmed/8696078/

Citrate undermines the Ferroxidase activity of Cp which is ESSENTIAL for scores of biological functions, not the least of which is regulating the use of Iron in the body... I'm just starting to assess this further, and will be writing a Post and Blog later re this...

I've loooooong poo-pooed citrate as that molecule is irritating to the bowel. However, I've just recently come to learn how "D"evastating it is to Ceruloplasmin and its VITAL Ferroxidase activity. It's mind-numbing, truth be known...

The Citrate molecule has a powerful relationship with Iron. And as we're learning, Iron may NOT be all its been cracked up to be!

COPPER: – OOPS WE DID IT AGAIN

Three KEY Oxidants; therefore Reduced Oxidative Species (ROS):

o   Superoxide, $\bullet O_2-$
o   Hydrogen Peroxide, H_2O_2
o   Hydroxyl Radical, $\bullet OH$(with an attitude...)

Three KEY SOD's (Superoxide Dismutases)

o   SOD1 = Intracellular CuZn SOD (Copper is catalytic, Zn is structural)

o   SOD2 = Mitochondria MnSOD

o   SOD3 = Extra cellular CuSOD

All Three Anti-Oxidant Enzymes have a NEED for Copper:

o   CuZnSOD

o   GSH (helps to recycle GSH via glutathione Peroxidase...)

o   Catalase (Yes, it's billed as Iron-dependent, but Iron ONLY work s when Copper is bio-available!...)

The more "proper" Copper, the greater the potential to make Cp. However, if that individual is a total "Stress!" Cadet, and has raging Stress hormones (ACTH >> Cortisol...) the machinery of the Cp production slows/stops... And that's a fact...

Also, if there's a toxic intake of "D"-only supplements, Calcium supplements, Iron supplements, HFCS, Glyphosate (Roundup), excess Rx meds, food additives, etc. and/or TOO LITTLE Maggie to spit at -- at least as how I'm seeing it -- "proper" Copper is a fine Stradivarius, but you STILL need a bow (Cp) to make it work!...

And as I noted earlier this am, making ATP is only HALF the issue. If the body lacks sufficient Mg to ATTACH to the ATP molecule, then the body can NOT recognize it, NOR can it use it. Mg-ATP is the key molecule for cellular energy...

That's been well chronicled, studied and suppressed since the 1920's...

Hopefully, that clarifies the point. I'm delighted beyond belief that we have access to a better form of Copper supplements, but there's STILL work to be done on the Liver and "Stress!" machinery...

The implication from MitoSynergy (http://mitosynergy.com) is that this is a supplement for ALL...

The 40 years of nutritional balancing that's been practiced at ARL and TEI Labs suggests that direct Copper supplements only works for ~20% of the population (Fast) and that the other 80% (Slow) is BETTER off with an indirect approach -- i.e. Wholefood Vit-C complex. (NOT Ascorbic Acid, mind you...)

But that may be "old" thinking, re: Copper supplementation... I simply don't know, at this point...

I'm quite confident that animal sources of Copper, i.e. Liver and other organ meats, are in a Cuprous format, in large part due to their likely being bound to Ceruloplasmin (Cp)...

This idea that ONLY plants produce Cuprous forms of Copper, in my humble opinion, is a bit misleading...

Andre Voisin's book, "Soil, Grass, Cancer" chronicled the LACK OF COPPER circa 1957 -- two generations BEFORE our current crisis. The late 1950's was a time BEFORE the hyper-assault of commercial fertilizers, not to mention the end-stage mechanisms of today's world to LOWER bioavailable Copper:

o   Glyphosate...(Round Up)
o   HFCS... (High Fructose Corn Syrup)
o   Vaccines...

Also, leading Copper researchers (Loren Pickart, PhD, among others) would suggest that our daily RDA of Copper SHOULD be closer to 6-8 mgs/day -- an amount that the conventional dietary world would find TOXIC!...

ALL is NOT as it seems...

We are animals, too... and they need "proper" Copper just as much as we do...

I'm just challenging this "PC," "Go Green!" belief that plants are the ONLY workhorses in making and sourcing "proper" Copper...

It doesn't make sense to me...

But I could be ALL wet here... (Don't think I am, however...)
What I have noted in the last 7 years of working with and interacting with LOTS of (2,500+) chronically ill folks:

o   MOST eat Smoothies for breakfast...
o   MOST (all but 6 out of 2,500 clients) are REPULSED by
        the thought of eating Liver... (Genelle included)

Hmmmmmmm...

While I have no "proof" of this, Copper from animals will be bound to Cp... Copper from veggies is unbound. And, parenthetically, I see no reason why Liver use would "distort" the upcoming blood test...

Again, I'm unaware of any restrictions prior to these tests...
Highest concentration of Cu(Cp?):

o   Organ meats...
o   Oysters...
o   Shellfish...
o   Perch...

Yummmmmmm...

Folks, please keep this in mind...

Because it appears that the Methyltransferase enzymes are activated with Copper -- NOT an insignificant fact, by the way... -- when the "Genes stop working..."

It APPEARS "genetic," when, IN FACT, it is a generational dysfunction of Copper metabolism that is passed from one minerally dysfunctional placenta to the next generation...

It is MOST subtle, but MOST effective...

This process of mineral depletion/ exorcism in our soils and foods has been working flawlessly for the last 75 years to the point that now we have an entire generation that believes that they are "genetically broken..." when the issue might be the pervasive nature of Mercury to bind up and destroy the effectiveness of this KEY mineral, we know as Copper!!...

All is NOT as it seems... that much I know!...

Is there any way to restore the lost myelin sheath, we would be the RATS in this study...

http://www.ncbi.nlm.nih.gov/pubmed/1252145

Take Mo' Wholefood Vit-C Complex... NOT Ascorbic Acid...

Before everyone runs out to "D"ump their bodies of the booga-wooga Copper, please step back and put the lens of Ceruloplasmin on that wonderful book...

From my conversations with Ann Louise Gittleman, the next version of that book will be VERY different, as the concept of "Copper deficiency" was not well understood.

My point, I was reading a text on Copper metabolism given to me by Teddie Miller (Thanks, again!) and one of the authors very clearly stated, *"the symptoms of Copper excess and Copper deficiency are almost identical..."*

That statement confirms my concept of "Cu-nundrum!" which is:

o   Too little usable Copper... AND
o   Too much unusable Copper existing simultaneously in
         our cells, our tissues and our bodies...

BOTH OF WHICH ARE THE RESULT OF TOO LITTLE Cp (Ceruloplasmin) and TOO MUCH BELIEF IN THE "D"IETARY "D"ICTUMS OF Mainstream Medicine and Mainstream Nutrition...

The supplement MSM, is really good at lowering Copper... But it takes between 6-8 Copper ions (they're still debating this...) to MAKE 1 molecule of Cp...

It's all a matter of balance, but most folks go overboard on supplements, including MSM...

At the risk of tugging on your cape...

The issue here is NOT Copper.

THE issue is the body's ability to produce the protein, Ceruloplasmin (Cp) which is ESSENTIAL to make BOTH Copper and Iron usable in the body. And its role in Iron metabolism is staggering, particularly in light of sooooo little attention given to it.

I'm new to this process of wellness coaching and have only done ~2,500 HTMAs in the last 7 years, but I've also evaluated several hundred Blood tests for clients in the last year. What I can assure you is that the term "Copper deficiency" is a complete misnomer...

There is a RAGING "Ceruloplasmin deficiency," and its lack in our bodies is the source of MUCH malaise due to:

o   Lack of bioavailable Copper...

o   Excess of bioUNavailable Copper...

o   Excess of bioUNavailable Iron (It's called "Iron Overload" in the literature...)

o   Imbalances galore with Zinc, and Manganese and countless metabolic pathways...

It's time we call a spade, a spade and help folks around the Globe know what the REAL battle ground is...

While technically Zinc is a Copper antagonist, the antagonism is very weak, based on intracellular analysis it only inhibits Copper absorption in the intestines.

Once Copper is absorbed, zinc seems to have little effect. The big Copper antagonists are chromium, sulfur, and ascorbic acid (not to be confused with the wholefood vitamin C complex),

61

followed by molybdenum and nickel.

Low chromium, low sulfur, and high aluminum are often the usual suspects in high Copper, but chromium should only be supplemented when calcium, Magnesium, and potassium are within normal range.

The most common cause of high unbound Copper is excessively high Copper levels, which can often benefit from sulfur sources, which interferes with Copper storage (sources include eggs, onion, garlic, MSM, taurine, NAC, and glucosamine sulfate [caution: glucosamine sulfate may raise blood sugar]).

Let's be sure to keep one thing in mind re Copper and ATP...

MOST who are sucking wind re "proper" Copper are chronically "Stressed Out!" and their Livers lack the natural mojo to make Ceruloplasmin (Cp), a KEY antioxidant enzyme of its own right...

This coupled with the fact that "Stress!" DEPLETES Mg -- it's how we're wired as a species. And ATP without Mg DOES NOT WORK. ATP MUST have that mineral to be functional inside the cell. Magnesium influences ATP in 3 profound ways:

1)   To change its stereochemical structure...
2)   Change its valence (-4>>-2) from 4- to 2-)
3)   Change its electromagnetic viability inside the cell...

In my world, Maggie and proper Copper are the Conductor (Mg) and 1st Violin (Cu) of the mineral Orchestra INSIDE our cells... They are BOTH essential to make beautiful music, and note that a violinist is LOST without her/his bow, yet Copper is "lost" without Cp...

62

I think it is safe to say, the more "proper" Copper, the greater the potential to make Cp in their livers. However, if that individual is a total "Stress!" Cadet, and has raging Stress hormones (ACTH >> Cortisol...) the machinery of the Cp production slows/stops...

And that's a fact...

I find the following intriguing;

o   Copper is essential for energy production in the Mitochondria to activate Complex IV to make ATP (via cytochrome c oxidase)...

o   Copper is essential for proper methylation... there are ~200 methyltransferase enzymes, and while I've only studied 10 CAREFULLY, Copper was required in all 12... I'm assuming the rest are to...

o   L-carnitine, CoQ10 and B-Vitamins ALL require methylation, to work properly...

MAJOR Hmmmmmmmmm...
And guess what mineral MOST folks have LOW bioavailable amounts of?...

You guessed it!...

Copper, especially "proper Copper," ie. Bio-available Copper.

The Thymus gland, part of the Lymphatic System is a Copper-rich gland... In studies of creating Copper-deficient RATS, it is well documented that the Spleen and Thymus are DRAMATICALLY affected by a lack of Copper...

Here's a study by Roger Prohaska, PhD, one of the world's authorities on Copper and the notable impact of Copper deficiency on mammals:

http://jn.nutrition.org/content/113/8/1583.full.pdf

Please up your Mg intake... this study will likely make your toes curl, an obvious sign of excessive MBR (Mg Burn Rate...)

The FLIP-side to this dynamic is to assess Iron "deficiency" status. More often than not, in my humble opinion, Iron dysregulation has LITTLE to do with Iron, and EVERYTHING to do with Ceruloplasmin (Cp) status...

And if Cp is weak, it's a safe bet that Cu,ZnSOD is weak, thus the body's innate Anti-Oxidant Enzyme defense system is weak...

And if SOD is weak, it's a safe bet that there's excess, unbound Iron that's CREATING an Oxidative Storm and ALL that "Oxidative Stress!" (That we KNOW as Rust...) is RAPIDLY aging the Thymus, other glands and organs, and the body overall...

Copper supplements in a "SLOW" Oxidizer -- ~80% of Society -- are NOT a good supplement option... Yes, everything about restoring Copper/Ceruloplasmin metabolism is counter-intuitive...

Also, you might find it fascinating that the "Red Nucleus" of the brain, is bordered on either side by the Substantia Nigris. And what is the "Red Nucleus" composed of, Hemoglobin and Ferritin...

The healthier the levels of Cp, the healthier the balance of both Hemoglobin and Ferritin... Said another way, the LOWER the Cp in this key section of the brain, the MORE dysfunctional these two KEY Iron proteins will be...

And Cp is ESSENTIAL to manage the flow of Iron between the two...

Guess what's required to convert retinoic acid from retinol?.....

Zinc!!!

Hmmmmm...

Doesn't SOD need zinc too??

To make 13-cis Retinoic Acid, which is what ACTIVATES the production of Ceruloplasmin, the body MUST have Copper...

There are THREE forms of SOD...

Yes, it does take a village, and of course Zinc is important. My intent, however, it to CHALLENGE the knee-jerk training that we have ALL received to view Zinc as the HERO and Copper (and Ceruloplasmin) as the VILLAIN...

It is anything but, and there is a "D"earth of practitioners who TRULY understand and act on that reality...

My focus re these issues is to challenge the blind assertion that Zinc will "solve" a Copper issue. I am sincerely trying to learn how that's the answer, and as was noted ^^^, it is about balance, and in MTHR NATURE, the critical nutrients, found in food, like Zinc and Copper and Iron are found TOGETHER as they are in Liver...

A very common mistake in the world of convention is to fixate on Copper and Zinc, and ignore COMPLETELY the status of

Ceruloplasmin (Cp) and the many parts of Iron metabolism -- WHICH are JOINED at the hip!

All too often, practitioners are "blinded" by the excess, unbound Copper, have no metric on Cp, only measure Ferritin (which is akin to TSH for Thyroid function...), see that the Zn/Cu ratio is "TOO LOW," recommend Zinc supplementation, and are unaware that that simple and ON THE SURFACE clinically-defendable act, is actually preventing the proper production of Cp in the Liver due to Zinc's powerful effect on restricting Copper absorption and thus Copper metabolism in the Liver...

This was recently highlighted in the following study:

http://jcp.bmj.com/content/68/9/723

Hope that clarifies the dynamic, as least as I've come to understand it...

https://ntischool.com/2015/06/dr-richard-olree-on-minerals-for-the-genetic-code-part-1/

Fat is KEY to proper Copper absorption...

Zinc is a very popular supplement, but it easily SHUTS DOWN Ceruloplasmin production in the Liver. Caution and Cp clarity are KEY to this process...

As I delve deeper and deeper into the TRUE source of metabolic dysfunction, the ORIGIN of our collective woes is Iron-induced Oxidative Stress. Period. And the CAUSAL agent for Iron mismanagement is a LACK OF CERULOPLASMIN... Kept firmly in check by the raging "D"ementia worldwide.

Also, the HTMA is most revealing as the level of Iron -- invariably shows LOW -- is revealing the USABLE level of Iron, and by inference, the level of Cp...

Lack of Bioavailable Copper to provide KEY Anti-Oxidant Enzymes (SOD, CAT, GSH) and Excess, unmanaged Iron that creates Oxidative Stress (ROS) are flip sides of the same Ceruloplasmin coin...

Ceruloplasmin REQUIRES Retinol, (animal-based Vitamin-A) among many other factors...

Hormone-D, taken in ANY supplemental form -- WITHOUT 10X the Retinol -- PREVENTS PROPER BALANCE OF RETINOL IN YOUR LIVER...

Based on my reading of the research and sxperience with clients, the "D" in that "D"emonic supplement stands for:

o   "D"estruction...
o   "D"isease...
o   "D"eath...

No "D"oubt about "D"at... ;-)

IRON: FACTORS TO CONSIDER

RBCs (Red Blood Cells) last for ~120 days when Copper is sufficient.

When Cu deficient, these cells LOSE 100 days of life!...

This has HUGE implications for creating energy from Oxygen-starved Haemoglobin...

Anemia is when your red blood cells are dying BEFORE they expire, due to lack of support - Ceruloplasmin is the transporter of the protein that supports red blood cells....

So support Ceruloplasmin, to support your red blood cells....

http://www.mdpi.com/2072-6643/5/7/2289/htm

It's one of my favorites! It really helps explain the interplay between Copper enzymes and the regulation of Iron...

It would be on the "Day 1" Reading List for Mg Man's Med School!...

Here's a MUST read by Kate Clancy who de-bunks the popular MYTH that women engaged in menses will have/develop "Iron-deficient anemia..."

http://blogs.scientificamerican.com/context-and-variation/httpblogsscientificamericancomcontext-and-variation20110727Iron-deficiency-anemia/

Nothing could be FUUUUURTHER from the truth. If your doctor truly believes that being female = IDA (Iron Deficiency Anemia), that may be a focal point for re-assessing whether that is a relationship that has your best interest at heart... or is there metabolic truth to their belief system....

The more I read and the more I learn about Iron OVERLOAD –
CAUSED by lack of bioavailable Copper (due to lack of
Ceruloplasmin!...) – the more convinced I am that this
misunderstanding of mineral metabolism is at the base of MOST,
if not ALL, chronic diseases… Iron dysregulation has profound
implications for Mg, Copper. Calcium, Estrogen, Thyroid
Function, etc…

I assure you, there will be MORE on this "Iron-ic" topic later, but
for now, please come to better understand that your doctor's
initials now seems to stand for "Meme Dispenser!"

Hope you find Kate Clancy's blog/article as enlightening as I did
this morning…

Again, as I have noted time, and time, and time again – we are,
indeed, being MISLED and being MSFED….

**There is not ONE aspect of Iron dysfunction that is NOT
caused by Copper dysregulation.**

The HINGE between these key minerals is Ceruloplasmin (Cp). It
takes EIGHT (8) Copper ions to make ONE Ceruloplasmin
molecule...

Cp is THE factor for making sure that:

o   Iron gets absorbed properly via Hephaestin...

o   Iron gets INTO Transferrin for proper transport...

o   Iron gets INTO Hemoblobin for optimal Oxygenation of
       the blood

o   Iron gets INTO/OUT OF Ferritin for optimal storage of a
       TOXIC form of Iron

o   Iron is properly regulated by the hormone, Hepcidin, as it takes bioavailable Copper/Ceruloplasmin to do so...

That conventional medicine is "SILENT" about this, or worse yet, UNAWARE of these foundational mineral dynamics -- worldwide -- should send a *chill* down everyone's back...

In the extensive reading and research that I've done re the Cu<>Fe interdependence, there is NO SUCH THING as "Iron anemia..." That is PURE "D"eception and "D"isinformation. As far back as the 1860's, it was acknowledged that "Iron Anemia" was due to Copper bioavailability.

Sorry to be so blunt, but the scale of this alleged "Iron" issue is due to a lack of proper understanding HOW the human body uses and relies on Ceruloplasmin to make BOTH Copper and Iron usable in the body...

Scientists have KNOWN this truth since 1928. That's the 1st reference that I've found about these mineral dynamics... It's time for that mystery to end and I applaud Kate Clancy for her enterprising work to pull back this curtain as billions of women around this Globe are being MISLED and MISFED...
Sorry to drop that bomb and NOT explain it more fully...

Copper is, indeed, key to the activation of the enzyme needed to make Estrogen... And when Copper is NOT so "proper," (i.e. lack of the KEY anti-oxidant, Ceruloplasmin...) it gets bound to Estrogen as it, too, is an anti-oxidant...

So, what's the connection to Iron?... Please review this article:

http://www.ncbi.nlm.nih.gov/pmc/articles/PMC3380187/pdf/12263_2012_Article_293.pdf

There are many switch-backs in that study, but suffice it to say that Estrogen has an effect on Hepcidin which affects Iron metabolism. I've NOT sorted this entire mechanism out, as

Hepcidin works best with proper Copper, and I'm just now getting my head around the Estrogen >> Hepcidin >> Ferroportin angle...

Iron metabolism is ENTIRELY dependent on bioavailable Copper and Ceruloplasmin that are NEVER assessed by Allopathetic practitioners who are obsessed by Iron "deficiency," are trained to "attack" Copper toxicity and IGNORE Copper toxicity...

(Were I a conventional type, I would, too, to ENSURE a waiting room full of sick and dysfunctional patients!...)

This requires a VERY different mindset and diagnostic approach to get to the TRUTH of this condition...

Beware the "Mintraps!" (mineral traps)... Low ALP means low RELATIVE Zinc to excess, unbound Copper...

Driving your Ferritin to the Moon affects your Liver's ability to make Ceruloplasmin (Cp). BOTH your Iron and Copper become UNusable, Oxidative Stress! rises, and ALP increases as a result.

The KEY to addressing these confusing mineral dynamics?

Focus on Ceruloplasmin production and STOP trying to out-think your Liver...

There are 10 "STOPs" and 10 "STARTs"... Wholefood Vit-C is but ONE Start... CLO is another Start... (*please refer to Ceruloplasmin Chapter for more details.*)

Now that we know about the different values of Copper Cu1 and Cu2 and the health impact of that, is there a similar situation with Iron or other minerals? Taking zinc long term to detox Copper can cause a reduction in Iron unbioavailabity, but is fixing it more complicated than just taking an Iron pill? Is there more than one form of Iron?

Yes, there are two principle forms of Iron, "proper" (Fe2+) as Charles Barker would likely say, and TOXIC (Fe3+) as I like to say.

There are SEVEN aspects to Iron Metabolism:

1)   Dietary Intake

2)   Intestinal Absorption

3)   Mineral Transport

4)   Metabolic use (principally for Heme-based proteins and enzymes, as well as Iron<>Sulfur Clusters)

5)   Storage (for the most part, Ferritin and this is Fe3+ -- it has the potential to become a TOXIC form of Iron! This "obsession that many have with Mo' Ferritin do NOT understand it's NON-METABOLIC role in the body...)

6)   Recycling of Iron (mostly in the Reticuloendothelial System) involving the spleen, the kidneys and the bone marrow.

7)   Epithelial Excretion (1-2 mg/day)

And through these seven stages, Iron is BOUNCING from 2+ >> 3+ >> 2+ >> 3+... It's amazing, actually...

Now here's where it gets FASCINATING...

ALL of those stages are dependent on Ceruloplasmin (Cp), which is a KEY anti-oxidant enzyme that has "Ferroxidase" properties...

That's a fancy way of saying that Iron is TOXIC without Cp!...

Or said another way, our bodies get "rusted" when Iron is without Cp...

Why?...

It is a guarantee that our level of Oxidative Stress will RISE due to excess, unbound Iron...

(It's worth noting that each molecule of Cp has FOUR Proper [1+] Coppers, and FOUR not-so-proper [2+] Coppers with an Oxygen molecule complete in the center...)

Cp, given its CENTRAL role to make IRON SAFE and USABLE, makes it one of the MOST important proteins/enzymes in the human body, in my humble opinion.

It is rather alarming that MOST, if not ALL, conventional doctors are unaware of its connection to BOTH Copper and Iron, are unaware of its oxidative role in the body, and NEVER measure its status when looking into Iron issues...

Based on my reasearch and experience, there is "NO fix" attached to taking Iron supplements. That is a HOAX being perpetrated on an unsuspecting public by practitioners that are CLUELESS about the TRUTH of Copper and Iron Metabolism, and their dependance on Ceruloplasmin.

My focus is SQUARELY on helping clients build up their Ceruloplasmin status, and IGNORE the histrionics and mythology of Zinc and Iron...

It seems to be working, especially given the fact that, once again, it is in DIRECT opposition to conventional thought... And yes, it is more than "a simple pill..." There are 20+ Steps in the process to enable the Liver to make optimal levels of Ceruloplasmin -- these are in the files of this page and the MAG page, as well...

In response to an inqury by a MAG-pie: *Why would someone who has good Iron levels but poor ferritin levels and feel better when taking Iron supplements?*

Your Cp is stronger than 98% of the clients I work with, coupled with a high serum Copper...

That said, your Zinc is ~75% of Ideal, and I've only got one Iron marker -- besides Ferritin which is VERY LOW -- so I'm not sure about that aspect of the Zn<>Cu<>Iron triangle. And we're only now addressing your Mn, which is now 6% of Ideal, and that plays a KEY role in supporting Iron metabolism...

My guess is that it has something to do with low Mn and too much serum Copper... As we all know, it is dangerous to "generalize" and folks like you exist to keep us humble and searching for MORE answers...

The OTHER side to this critical Cp molecule is the role that it plays in response to Inflammation...

And yes, Cp will RISE under those conditions, as well as in response to infection, pregnancy and the use of birth control pills...

And what we don't know is what is the status of your CRP (C-Reactive Protein) that is the most sensitive marker for Inflammation. We have yet to get a Mag RBC for you, and know that Maggie and CRP ride on a seesaw together...

It is possible that your Mg is low, that your CRP is high, which is WHY your Cp is elevated and that is causing Iron to be diverted from Ferritin to AVOID allowing its access to pathogens...

If, indeed, that is the case of an infection/inflammation, "feeding" your body Iron would be the LAST thing you would want to do...

That's a whole other side to Cp and it's difficult to know which playing field we're in just based on limited markers that we typically work with...

Ideally, it requires a more complete mineral profile and blood test to properly answer your excellent question.

THE ultimate metabolic issue is the Liver's ability to produce Cp...

What is still in the "not sure" state for me is to what extent "proper Copper" ensures the optimal production of Cp...

I've identified 18 steps, and counting, that get in the way. Even the BEST of Copper supplements can NOT overcome the lunacy of some supplements, like hypervitaminosis D that absolutely gets in the way...

In my humble opinion, using Ferritin to assess "Iron status" is the equivalent of using TSH to assess Thyroid status. It is a flawed, misleading and lazy approach to assessing what's REALLY going on metabolically. The fact that Allopathetic practitioners use this should cause you to pause.....

To understand Iron, these are the markers to assess:

o   Hemoglobin

o   Hematocrit count

o   Serum Ceruloplasmin (it protects Iron and Copper!)

o   Serum Iron

o   Serum Transferrin

o   Serum TIBC (% SAT)

o   Serum Copper

o   Plasma Zinc

o   Mag RBC

The most OVERLOOKED reason for LOW Iron is the likely presence of a bacterial infection and low Ferritin is the body's wisdom to PREVENT the bacteria having access to Fe to accelerate their growth...

And the "you need TONS of Iron for good Thyroid function," is ALSO misleading... You need TONS of bioavailable Copper to MAKE THAT IRON USABLE...

Please start questioning the conventional "D"ogma and "D"iagnostic parameters... They are NOT designed to improve your health and wellbeing!

http://www.alzforum.org/news/research-news/Iron-export-new-role-links-app-metals-oxidative-stress

That's one of my favorite articles to reveal the profound importance of Copper to having bioavailable Iron. They are Siamese twins with Ceruloplasmin (Cp) as their bridge... Far more interdependent than most realize...

Metals can be most disruptive, and despite what many may be thinking about Mercury, Iron is a MAJOR source of metabolic dysfunction and disruption that we OFTEN overlook...

We are conditioned to think we need COPIOUS amounts of Iron and its overload is WILDLY disruptive to the body... as is Copper. Both Copper and Iron -- when NOT bound to their protein Ceruloplasmin -- are MOST disruptive to the mechanics and metabolism of the body...

Leading Cardiologists have a VERY different view of "optimal" Ferritin... THEIR Functional Range is 20-50 mg/dL...

Why?...

Because they know that as the Ferritin level rises above 50, the risk of Heart Attacks and Heart Events gets stratospheric... It calls to question the OBSESSION that many have with trying to get their Ferritin to between 80-100... It makes about as much sense as seeking to get one's Cholesterol to 0...

o   Haphaestin is a KEY Iron protein designed to grab dietary Iron and put it in the blood stream. It is ACTIVATED by Copper that is found at the CORE of the wholefood Vit-C molecule...

o   Ceruloplasmin (Cp) is ALSO involved in this process, and it, TOO, is Copper dependent as 6-8 Copper ions are ESSENTIAL to make 1 molecule of Ceruloplasmin...

o   Iron without Cp is ROGUE... pure and simple!...

Iron Supplementation WITHOUT commensurate Ceruloplasmin (Ferroxidase, for those Iron-ophile researchers out there...) production from the Liver to handle it and metabolize it will CREATE Oxidative Stress!...

And that's a scientific fact...

"Hair Loss" is a classic response to "Stress!" >> Mg Loss >> Copper dysregulation >> Loss of Cp production >> Increase of Toxic Iron>>increase of ROS>> that affects metabolic pathways...

MOST forms of Liver have a higher concentration of Copper over Iron and Zinc, believe it or not...

Anemic Ceruloplasmin makes for anemic Ferritin. That latter Iron protein does NOT respond to Iron supplements! That coupled with the anemic level of Mg (the MAG Ref Range STARTS at 5.0-7.0 mg/dL) means you're ~ "2 quarts low"... And you and I both know you'd NEVER drive your car out of the gas station without filling the engine with oil, if the dipstick in fact, showed you were "2 quarts low"...

Right?...

There clearly are residual issues with the Mercury dynamic that are playing out in your body... The obvious issue is that your mineral foundation is imbalanced and it's affecting numerous metabolic pathways...

What's KEY in this process is to acknowledge that a "Copper issue" is NEVER just about Copper and, in fact, has an impact on other metals and minerals... For Example:

o   Yes, your Usable Copper is near ideal @ 98.1 ("Ideal" = 100)

o   Yes, your Unusable Copper is @ 27.9%, but many of my clients are 2X that level... ("Ideal" = 10-15%)

o   Yes, his Ceruloplasmin is -- again -- near Ideal @ 32.7 ("Ideal" = 33)

So let's FIRST acknowledge the significance of that... Huge shifts in KEY blood markers -- that relate to KEY Metabolic Enzymes activated by Copper... -- that Mineral Denialists NEVER even talk about...

The importance of Cupro-enzymes, especially the enzyme, Ceruloplasmin (Cp), in the OPTIMAL functioning of Homo Normalus is akin to comparing Mt. Everest to the metabolic molehills that most practitioners obsess over...

Now, what's still "off-kilter" with his latest blood panel?...

o   Perhaps your Zinc is 60% HIGHER than Ideal ("Ideal = ~110)... and

o   Perhaps your Ferritin is 90, and while leading Endocrinologists and Thyroid groups will sing Hozana to that level, leading Cardiologists are STRONGLY advising their patients that the optimal Ferritin Functional Range = 20-50 mg/dL, and that levels above 50 CAUSE an uptick of heart events... (All this based on a KEY study in Finland in 1992...)

And why is that elevated Iron issue so important? Well, Ferritin is a storage protein for UNUSABLE Iron.

Hmmmmm...

WHY are we exalting a storage protein for UNUSABLE Iron?... That is the form of Iron that when it gets into the cell, CAUSES Oxidative Stress (we know this process as RUST)...

That is NOT good, as MOST chronic conditions are the RESULT of unchecked Oxidative Stress INSIDE the cell and INSIDE the tissues...

The research is increasingly CLEAR, this "RUST" is brought to us by Iron Overload and Copper deficiency because of their respective impact on Reactive Oxygen Species (Iron) and Anti-Oxidant Enzymes (Copper)....

So, I don't think that you have a Copper issue...

I'm more concerned with the Ferritin level and the effect that THAT might be having on his unusable Copper dynamic... And the elevated Zinc is also curious, which we've got to address, as well...

The Blessing and Curse of Mineral Balancing is the endless wheels of interaction that these amazing catalytic agents engage in that DIRECTLY affect the functionality of our metabolism, via our Enzymes.

And the true TRAGEDY of our contemporary society is that Allopathetic Mineral Denialists are an embarrassment to our intellect and our integrity, In my humble opinion, because they are CLUELESS about my blah, blah, blah outlined above^^^...

I'm STILL trying to get my head around this IRON-Y that I just pieced together:

WHY is the world is convention "training us" -- like Circus Bears -- to focus on a protein (Ferritin) that STORES ~20% of Iron in the body IN AN UNUSABLE FORMAT, And Teaching us to IGNORE the KEY Iron protein (Hemoglobin) that carries 70% of Iron is a TOTALLY USABLE FORMAT?!?...

And, to add to that mystery, WHY do they NEVER measure Ceruloplasmin status, given that it's ALSO called Ferroxidase enzyme (in Iron Research Labs around the world...) which is ESSENTIAL to make turn Ferric Iron (3+) >> Ferrous Iron (2+) so that is can be USED IN METABOLIC TRANSACTIONS?...

Yet another twist and FURTHER evidence that Allopathetic Medicine is Affagato!....

In my humble opinion, I would stay FAAAAAR away from supplemental Iron. The combo of wholefood Vit-C + Black Strap Molasses appears to be a blockbuster way to elevate restore Iron function...

As I'm digging into this issue, it's VERY clear that the world of convention (doctors and nutritionists) have it PERFECTLY backwards,– AGAIN! – when it comes to correcting issues related to the Iron proteins and Iron metabolism...

And the acid test question for you is: what is your Ceruloplasmin status?!?... If you don't know, you're wasting your time. It is the KEY to Iron metabolism. And for those that get entertained by abject absurdity, this enzyme is ALSO called Ferroxidase to Iron researchers...

Heaven forbid they agree on a naming nomenclature that wouldn't confuse the world trying to "solve" their Iron issues because their Copper metabolism is hopelessly tweaked by conventional practitioners who are also CLUELESS about Copper and its metabolic supremacy un hundreds of critical enzymes!...

THE issue is your Ceruloplasmin status... Ferritin is DEPENDENT on that protein!...

Let me try once more....

The over-riding conclusion following 6 months of intensive reading and research re Iron:

"Iron anemia -- in ALL its forms -- is a clinical sign of Copper deficiency." Period!

Please note, I've actually read that in 2 different stuffy, peer-reviewed studies... No, I didn't remember to record the exact citation for the doubting Thomases who are ready to pounce!...

The EARLIEST recorded documentation of this TRUTH re Iron<>Copper dynamic, is 1862!... (Sorry, that ain't a typo!)

PLEASE FORGET ABOUT THE IRON...

It takes 8 atoms of Copper to make 1 molecule of Ceruloplasmin...

Focus on your COPPER, Ceruloplasmin and the Iron will take care of itself...

Here is the study that I used, it is all about how even rats with high Iron levels were anemic due to Copper deficiency. It's a little heavy but is excellent reading.

http://jn.nutrition.org/content/103/2/196.full.pdf

That is one of my favorite studies!...

You are NOW deemed Ambassador of Wholefood Vit-C and you have MY permission to take this helm and steer any future threads into the harbor of sanity and truth!...

Kudo's on your openness to the TRUTH and conviction to spread same in a setting of potential resistance (i.e. school...)
Iron metabolism is ENTIRELY dependent on bioavailable Copper and Ceruloplasmin, which are NEVER assessed by Allopathic practitioners who are "obsessed" by Iron deficiency, "attack" copper toxicity and IGNORE Ceruloplasmin...

(I would, too, to ENSURE a waiting room full of sick and dysfunctional patients!...)

These metal dynamics requires a VERY different mindset and diagnostic approach to get to the TRUTH of this condition...

This misunderstanding re Copper<>Iron is DEEPLY ingrained in the minds and practices of Allopathetics AND Alternatives alike!

I'll do what I can to assist, but please lower your expectations otherwise...

Please note: LOW Ferritin is NOT an Iron Issue...

It is AGGRAVATED by Iron supplements that SHUT DOWN Copper metabolism and the production of Ceruloplasmin...

I am a self-trained Mineral Detective that elected to become a wellness coach as I couldn't stand the INSANITY of the conventional system that I worked in for 32 years as an exec/consultant...

I ain't NO doctor, nor do I pretend to be one on TV, but I am TOTALLY committed to helping folks, especially MAG-pies, learn how their bodies REALLY work...

http://gotmag.org/work-with-us/

I believe this is the study worth looking at:

http://circ.ahajournals.org/content/86/3/803.full.pdf

That's ^^^ a pretty technical article, but here's a wonderful piece by Bill Sardi -- a very gifted health writer -- who will explain why EXCESS IRON AIN'T all it's cracked up to be...

http://knowledgeofhealth.com/revelation-statin-cholesterol-lowering-drugs-work-via-their-ability-to-reduce-iron-stores-not-cholesterol/

In this article, Sardi highlights the work of Leo R. Zacharski, MD who has discovered the IRON-LOWERING aspect of $tatin$ and advises patients to keep their Ferritin between 20-50 ng/mL. Turns out you'd be better off working with Leeches than $tatin$!!!

And the cherry on the top of this "Iron-ic" issue is this OUTSTANDING article on Iron Fortification that should make EVERYONE in the US, UK, and CANADA quake in their "rusty" boots:

http://freetheanimal.com/2015/06/enrichment-theory-everything.html

Hope that does the trick...

There's enough there to make even the most ardent skeptic think twice about what is REALLY going on with Iron...

And, of course, as you have further questions, please ask away!..

Once again, I'm BREAKING with convention to reveal that HIGH Ferritin is NOT a sign of optimal Iron metabolism, despite the chest-beating of Neurologists, Endocrinologist and Thyroid groups, across the internet.

I'm taking my nod from Cardiologists who are VERY aware of the TOXIC effect of EXCESS Iron -- especially that which is stored in Ferritin, and can be the stimulus for Reactive Oxygen Species (ROS)...

At the risk of being PERFECTLY blunt, the Thyroid Groups are clueless about the full metabolic dynamics of Ferritin in regulating Thyroid function.

At the end of the day, it's ALL about Ceruloplasmin (Cp), and its PROFOUND role to regulate EVERY FACET OF IRON METABOLISM.

Know that Cp contains EIGHT (8) atoms of Copper and IRON DON'T WORK properly without those Copper ions. In effect, Iron is the "Dummy" and Copper is the "Ventroliquist" telling it what to do...

By ALL means, please give up chasing the Iron dummy. But now shift your focus to the Metabolic Mag-ician of the body: Ceruloplasmin!...

Thyroid groups are SILENT on Ceruloplasmin and lack of Bioavailable Copper to MAKE SO-CALLED IRON ENZYMES work.

Again, it's not possible to answer a question about Ferritin in isolation of where the following are:

o **Mag RBC**
o **serum Copper**
o **serum Ceruloplasmin**
o **plasma Zinc**
o **serum Iron**
o **serum Transferrin**
o **serum TIBC (% Sat)**
o **serium Ferritin**

It is foolhardy, at best, to address that ONE marker and suggest you know the FULL metabolism of Iron in the body. It's akin to measuring TSH and saying you fully understand the functioning of the Thyroid. *TILT!!!* When practitioners try to do that, NOW! Righto?

THINGS THAT GO "BUMP" IN THE NIGHT...

My advice, grab your seatbelt... this is likely going to be a brief, bumpy, and bewitching ride...

As many of you know, I got into this wacky world of nutrition because I was convinced everyone simply had a Mg-deficiency -- thus was borne my wellness quest AND also exposed my nutritional/metabolic naiveté...

I have journeyed for the last 7 years to make sense of this mineral dynamics, with stops to better understand the dynamics of Na/K, Vitamin-D, Copper toxicity/dysregulation, and Ceruloplasmin metabolism... All was going reasonably well until the Universe dropped the Ace-in-the-Hole: Iron Overload...

And as I pursue this Rabbit-hole with a vengeance, I NOW realize WHY Magnesium is getting hosed, and WHY Copper is sooooo dysregulated. And the mechanics of understanding Oxidative Stress! and the role of Copper-dependent Anti-Oxidant enzymes (SOD, GSH [GSH-Px], and CAT) to STOP this "Rusting" process, and the role of Iron to CREATE Free Radicals (ROS) is legendary in the research labs around the globe.

OK, so where's he's going today?...

Here are four (4) articles that I invite ALL who are serious about re-gaining their health and metabolic equilibrium:

http://freetheanimal.com/2015/06/enrichment-theory-everything.html

http://jn.nutrition.org/content/134/11/3171S.full.pdf+html

http://circ.ahajournals.org/content/83/3/1112.full.pdf

https://www.researchgate.net/publication/26292763_Iron_and_M enopause_Does_Increased_Iron_Affect_the_Health_of_Postmen opausal_Women

If you take the time to read those article, which will keep you OFF the streets and FB for a good long while, what you'll SOON discover is that we're bring POISONED by Iron: in our food, properties of our water, Rx meds, vaccines, etc. The scale of it is mind-numbing to say the least.

For those that don't know Joseph McCord, PhD, he and his Advisor, Irwin Fridovich, PhD discovered SOD:

Superoxide Dismutase at Duke University in the late 1960's...

It is THE enzyme that is designed to neutralize the Superoxide radical (that's an Oxygen molecule with an attitude!...).

And as he points out in Equations #2 and #3 (known as the famous Haber/Weiss formula). In the absence of Copper-dependent SOD, it is a MAJOR source of ROS, especially the much-feared Hydroxyl Radical that causes SOOOO much destruction of lipids on the cell membrane and proteins and DNA within the cell...

And what's the gist of Jian et al (2009)?...

That group of enterprising researchers is taking a very different look at the aging process, especially the much discussed state of "Menopause!" Essentially, what they are challenging -- and appropriately so -- is that the core issues of this transition are equally related to Iron Overload, as they are to a lack of Estrogen...

That's a VERY different way of viewing Menopause, and the key conditions that are associated with this:

o   Hot Flashes...
o   Osteoporosis...
o   Skin Aging...

ALL of these conditions are brought to us by dysregulated Iron, courtesy of an organism that is swimming in bioUNavailable Copper and TOO LITTLE Ceruloplasmin, BOTH OF WHICH ARE ESSENTIAL for the proper regulation of ALL facets of Iron metabolism.

And folks who are chasing stratospheric levels of Ferritin, Calcium supplements, Fosamax, and HRT are apparently out of touch with what the leading research outlined ^^^^ is REALLY telling us... And when you factor in the Iron Fortification that is the underpinning of our grains, then it will REALLY hit home.

Rest assured, there will be more posts and threads on this topic -- I have NO doubt. This set of observations will cause rampant heartburn for all who take the time to read, reflect and re-evaluate their understanding of the "Aging" process. The Iron-y of this dynamic is captivating, just as any MAG-net is...

As always, I'll look forward to the blow-back and repartee that this will surely stimulate!...

Iron CAUSES the cell to LOWER its production of ATP...
Iron CAUSES the pH of the cell to become MORE Acidic...

Both ^^^ are PRE-REQUISITES for Fungus, that is already residing in our cells, to WAKE UP and do their functions...

And it is a WELL-ESTABLISHED fact that Fungus CAVES to E-SOD (found in RBC) and L-SOD (found in WBC)...

Fungus is a sign of mineral/metabolic mayhem, NOT the source of it...

In my humble opinion...

This is what occupied Louis Pasteur, MS and Antoine Beauchamp, MD, PhD (2), for decades!...

We've got miles to go, yet.....

It's taken me 12 weeks to sort this out, and I'm just on the headlines...

Fortified Flour is found in US, UK, and Canada, and THIRD WORLD COUNTRIES... The OTHER 72 nations of the "Western World" ban the fortification of flour -- for OBVIOUS reasons...

Chicken vs Egg phenomenon...

Again, keep in mind, the "System" wants us to "BELIEVE" that "D"isease comes 1st, and then metabolic mayhem follows... Hold a mirror up to their "D"ynamic and a VERY different picture emerges and the impact of certain dysregulated metals, i.e. Iron, become VERY important and VERY much the "D"river in these processes of infection and inflammation...

It's ALL about foreground Vs the field...

http://www.wellnessresources.com/weight/articles/stunning_disco veries_regarding_Iron_obesity_candida_thyroid/

OUTSTANDING article from a gifted nutritionist -- what a loss that he died on a routine jog...

In any event, two years earlier, Byron Richards, CCN, wrote about the seminal research of William Weglicki, MD, whose great contribution to science was that Mg deficiency is THE trigger for Inflammation:

http://www.wellnessresources.com/health/articles/Magnesium_is _essential_for_preventing_substance_p_overload/

The entire inflammatory cascade follows the cellular loss of Mg, that then triggers Substance P (which stands for "Production") and the inflammatory Cytokine Cascade is soon to follow.

89

Now it would make sense that under conditions of LOW Mg, i.e. Inflammation, the body would call upon Ceruloplasmin to respond, which it does:

http://www.ncbi.nlm.nih.gov/pubmed/4048245

Inflammation builds, and Cp plays a bigger role trying to sequester and regulate the excess Iron...

Now, here's an important article that profiles the regulatory role that Ceruloplasmin plays with Hepcidin. Yes, Hepcidin is a Hormone, but it takes its cues from Cp:

http://www.sciencedirect.com/science/article/pii/S092544391000 1481

No doubt, we won't resolve this "He said <> She said"...

It is a very important and subtle dynamic that underlies the metabolic process and how the body RESPONDS to "Stress-induced!" mineral loss and imbalance.

I firmly believe that the body has residing in it all the bugs and critters that can create problems, but they are naturally held in check by proper pH and energy levels, due to optimal levels and ratios of minerals that allow for the optimal functioning of metabolic and regulatory enzymes that RUN THE BODY and maintains homeostasis.

"Fungus is among us," but NOT because of an "infection" -- that is VERY outdated Allopathetic thinking (in my humble opinion), and fungus is ENTIRELY a dynamic that FOLLOWS the mineral imbalance, as noted in the seminal research of William Weglicki, MD, and the role of SOD to control fungus in the body.

That's a lot of blah, blah, blah... we just might need to record a conversation as we seek to sort all this out. And I very much look forward to that!...

Completely agree, but it is my understanding that it chelates the oxidized form of Copper (Copper II), therefore resveratrol's anti-cancer effects.

o   http://www.febsletters.org/article/S0014-5793(05)00570-3/abstract

o   http://www.ncbi.nlm.nih.gov/pubmed/15345806

o   http://www.ncbi.nlm.nih.gov/pmc/articles/PMC2615657/

o   http://www.greenmedinfo.com/article/curcumin-Iron-chelator-article-1

These are some GREAT articles...

So do you recommend avoiding cooking in cast Iron
I'm struggling with that question... and I know a couple of others have raised it...

What is a bit unsettling is that acidic foods cooked in an Iron Skillet raise the Iron content of the food several-fold. And steaming food in a cast Iron skillet does the SAME thing...

I'm still getting my head around this, and have used Iron skillets/pans my entire life.

I'm going to "punt" for now... I'll be back!

o   Iron for Women = 100 mg/dL
o   Iron for Men = 120 mg/dL
o   Ferritin = 20-50 mg/dL
(Per Leading Cardiologists)

The connection of glyphosate to Iron I realize this is "silent" on minerals:

http://www.gmoevidence.com/university-of-caen-roundup.../

I would suspect that the more recent practice of spraying wheat before harvest, allegedly to improve yield (*wink* *wink*...) is a major contributing factor. It is well documented that Glyphosate lowers Copper/raises Iron in the Liver. That is NOT a desirable state for hepatic metabolism...

At the risk of beating a "dead" horse...

"The underlying pathogenic event in Oxidative Stress is cellular Iron mismanagement."

(Thompson, K.I et al (2001) "Iron and Neurologic Disorders." Brain Research Bulletin, 55; 155-164)

For those seeking the granular TRUTH of how Iron is "MANAGED" inside our cells and inside our bodies:

o   Role of Cp on Iron regulation:
     http://www.ncbi.nlm.nih.gov/pmc/articles/PMC322742/pdf/j
     cinvest00228-0276.pdf
     (PAY PARTICULAR ATTENTION TO Fig. 6)

o   Role of Cp on Iron regulation in Copper deficient rats:
     http://jn.nutrition.org/content/103/2/196.full.pdf

o   Role on Cp on regulation of the Iron Hormone, Hepcidin:
     http://www.sciencedirect.com/science/article/pii/S0925443
     910001481

o   Role of Fe- and Cu-Homeostatic Mechanisms in Neuro-
     disorders:
     http://journal.frontiersin.org/article/10.3389/fphar.2012.001
     69/full

Please, step BACK from your misguided pursuits of Iron Loading to get your Iron storage protein, Ferritin, higher and higher, and reflect on what these contemporary studies are REALLY saying about the dangers or Iron and the MISMANAGEMENT of Iron.

All is NOT as you've been "prescribed...", nor as you've been trained to believe...

Researching that madly, on how we manage Iron overload....

o   Blood donations

o   Phytic Acid block Absorption, although it's not a sure-proof solution (see Mercola's article to that effect...)

o   Tannic Acids block Iron Absorption

o   Tumeric (Curcumin) has profound Iron-binding properties...

o   Sweating is an effective way to excrete Iron (Exercise and Infra-red lights)

o   The Herb, Rosemary, has recognized Iron blocking/binding affects

o   Activated Charcoal, although I'm still researching this...

o   Chemically, Desferroxiamine, is a recognized pharmaceutical agent for Iron binding

ANYONE with the Bookends of Iron Mis-management (#'s that are TOO LOW or TOO HIGH...) is WELL ADVISED to focus on optimal Ceruloplasmin production and function...

And yes, Liver, is STILL on my recommended list of Vittles to eat weekly to ensure optimal intake of B-Vitamins, correct balance of

Zn<>Cu<>Fe, molybdenum and 20,000 IUs of Retinol -- THE KEY Factor for synthesizing Ceruloplasmin...

Can Tumeric contribute to Iron anemia???

This is an important topic and appropriate question...

It may be a case of mistaken identity:

http://jn.nutrition.org/content/136/12/2970.full

I don't recall indicating that Tumeric can contribute to Iron anemia, it's possible, but it's not something that I would typically say.

That said, I do not routinely recommend Tumeric, largely because of the WIIIIIIIDE variation in quality and potency of this spice. Also, please note that it's NOT a part of my Ceruloplasmin protocol...

Let's hope that we can gain greater insights and understanding re this powerful nutrient and learn optimal ways of using it for our benefit...

I've assessed Cp in ~250 clients...

o   Functional Range is 25-40 mg/dL
o   Most are in the high teens/low 20's...
o   What I like folks to shoot for is ~35...

That said, Cp is considered an "Acute Phase Reactant..." It can get elevated when there's an inflammatory process infection, pregnancy or use of birth control pill, which can be triggered by excess, unbound Copper and/or Iron. And it makes perfect sense that it does, but if the Cp is elevated, you need to rule out Inflammation with a high sensitivity C-Reactive Protein (hsCRP) blood test.

Please read:

http://www.ncbi.nlm.nih.gov/pmc/articles/PMC3022063/pdf/jcbn-48-46.pdf

Once again, it's the BOOKENDS of Iron that will KILL your metabolism.

It is Ceruloplasim that REGULATES... the Iron proteins, that reduces Iron dysregulation....NOT INGESTING MORE IRON!

Iodine is necessary in Cp production, but please know that, my Iodine awareness is one of my glaring weaknesses... I have a very pedestrian understanding of this PROFOUNDLY important mineral. I believe that Guy Abraham, MD and his colleagues (Lynne Farrow, David Brownstein, MD, etc.) Are far better equipped to adress this Iodine.

I am still working to better understand how to address the iodine issue. There is a reason why it's LAST on this "How to restore Ceruloplasmin" list...

When the populous worldwide is being "D"rownned in Iron via "Fortification of Flour" (i.e. US, UK, Canada and many other "Third World" countries...) to what extent does THAT Iron Overload factor CAUSE this phenomenon noted in this article?...

Also, to what extent, given that Oxalates "chelate" metals, is this Oxalate phenomenon a PHYSIOLOGICAL REACTION to Excess Iron in the tissues of a rapidly increasing "magnetic" species?...

I'm TOTALLY on board with pursuing a Vulcan Mind-Meld!...

I'm coming to the conclusion that Oxalates are a by-product of a body that has rampant Copper<>Iron dysregulation and that this is an "evolutionary" response to Iron Overload...

That is based FAAAAR MORE on instinct, right now, as opposed

95

to compelling scientific proof...

Among the 3 GREATEST NUTRITIONAL LIES:

o   Calcium is GOOD for strong bones...
o   Cholesterol CAUSES Heart Disease...
o   Iron deficiency is the GREATEST mineral deficiency...

ALL 3 are PURE Social (Medical) Constructions of Reality to support a business model based solely on profit, NOT the person..

Here's my *dream* blood test outcome:

o   **Mag RBC = 6.0-6.5 mg/dL**

o   **Serum Ceruloplasmin = 33-35 mg/dL**

o   **Serum Iron = W: 100ug/dL // M: 120ug/dL**

o   **Serum TIBC = W: 285ug/dL // M: 340ug/dL**

o   **% Sat (Iron/TIBC) = 33%**

o   **Serum Ferritin = 20-50ng/mL (Please note, leading Cardiologists are sounding the ALARM re rising Ferritin levels and their connection to heart events...)**

These proposed values noted ^^^^ assume normal Hemoglobin and Hematocrit levels, which are predicated on optimal levels of bioavailable Copper, which is a function of optimal liver production of Ceruloplasmin...

You can NOT make Heme, you can NOT make Hemoglobin, and you can NOT load Iron into Hemoglobin (via the enzyme Ferrochelatase) WITHOUT optimal levels of Copper.

Please note, I have YET to see this *dream* profile in ANY client, to date... In large part because the System trained us -- like Circus Bears -- to demonize Copper and worship at the Altar of 'Mo Iron!

Again, it's a work in progress...

o   Ferrous (Fe++) Iron is an unstable form of Iron

o   Ferric (Fe+++) Iron is stable and is the state that Iron is Transported in...

o   To move from Fe++ >> Fe+++ requires Oxidation, which is the removal of ONE electron...

o   One of Ceruloplasmin's MOST IMPORTANT jobs is to Oxidize that Iron so that it can be properly loaded into Transferrin, as well as into the Iron Storage protein, Ferritin.

This FACT about Ceruloplasmin's REGULATORY role of Iron has been thoroughly researched and well known in RESEARCH circles since 1941. It is wonderfully depicted in Figure 6 of this article (found on pg 7). This is apparently NOT taught in Medical School... (You all can connect the dots on that obvious disconnect!)

http://www.ncbi.nlm.nih.gov/pmc/articles/PMC322742/pdf/jcinvest00228-0276.pdf

The object is NOT so much to deny our body of the Iron that is needs... but it is to focus on OPTIMIZING the production of Ceruloplasmin (Cp) production in the Liver and overcome the "D"in of "D"ietary "D"eception and "D"irectives that we have en"D"ured for the last 70+ years...

IRON ISSUES ARE NOT SOLVED BY INGESTING MORE IRON... THEY ARE SOLVED BY THE COPPER-DEPENDENT ENZYME, CERULOPLASMIN... as it REGULATES and affects the mechanics and optimization of Hephaestin, Transferrin, Ferroportin, Ferritin, and Hepcidin...

Period!

For those interested/worried about Alzheimer's and/or Parkinson's (AD/PD), this is a PROFOUNDLY important study -- from Iceland! -- clarifying the dynamics and significance of Ceruloplasmin (Cp) [in a good way...] and "Iron Stress!" [in a bad way].

http://www.ncbi.nlm.nih.gov/pmc/articles/PMC3493298/pdf/ndt-8-515.pdf

At the end of the day, Copper/Iron DYSREGULATION is at the epicenter of these vexing and destructive conditions that are a plague on society that is projected to become an epidemic in the coming decades. And the notion that we are: "Copper Toxic" and "Iron Deficient" is simply MORE EVIDENCE that we are living the psycho-drama of 1984! Where EVERYTHING is BACKWARDS!

ALL IS NOT AS IT SEEMS...

Please note, as I've said repeatedly and will continue to say..., these conditions are NOT medical disease... There are perfect signs of metabolic dysregulation brought about by mineral deficiencies (NOTE: Think LOW Bioavailable minerals...)

And lest you buy the BS re the booga-wooga "gene origin," KNOW that Iron Overload inside the cell CREATES •O2- (Superoxides!) that CAUSE DNA Damage. It is WELL chronicled in 1,000's of studies... Here's one that has been referenced 4,000+ times:

http://www.ncbi.nlm.nih.gov/pmc/articles/PMC1153442/pdf/biochemj00330-0011.pdf

And what NEUTRALIZES •O2-?...

Superoxide Dismutase -- CuZnSOD1 -- this VITAL Anti-Oxidant Enzyme is KEY to controlling the Oxidative Burden of run-away, mismanaged Iron that is CAUSED by a LACK OF Ceruloplasmin (Cp). And furthermore, SOD1, just like Cp is Copper DEPENDENT. (Zinc ^^^^ is purely structural in that SOD enzyme...)

Hope this study sheds new and important light on these two notable and other related Neurodegenerative conditions (ALS, MS, etc.). And please remember that our government mandates the fortification of Iron, AND has been doing so, since the beginning of World War II...

Please read, reflect and take appropriate action. You might also share this with your doctors so they, too, can learn this truth...What are the chances of undoing the damage?According to Jerry Tennant, MD (Dallas, TX), the ENTIRE CNS and Brain is rebuilt every 8 months!

Change the INPUTS and change the FUNCTION.

That's a long-winded way of saying: NO! It is NOT too late!

The PROBLEM is NOT UNDERSTANDING AND ACTING ON EXCESS Fe and TOO LITTLE Copper.

I do NOT know the effectiveness of DE (diatomaceous earth) here. Tumeric, however, is a recognized Iron chelator...

I would do this test to get to the TRUTH of your condition:

http://requestatest.com/mag-zinc-copper-panel-with-iron-panel-testing

You can ILL afford to put more Iron into a body that is STARVED for bioavailable Copper...

o   You can NOT make Heme without Copper...

o   You can NOT make Hemoglobin without Copper...

o   You can NOT INSERT Iron into the Hemoglobin without Copper to activate the KEY enzyme Ferrochelatase...

o   AND the degradation of Hemoglobin is EXCELERATED in a body that has LOW bioavailable Copper...

You might point ALL ^^^^ out to your doctor...

I'm still trying to sort out the BEST approaches... (It's intriguing that folks invariably want to blow past the PROFOUND importance of these kinds of research findings, AND IGNORE THE FACT that their doctors have had it ALL WRONG -- and have all along!... and simply cut to the chase of: "OK, so what do I do?!?"...)

I do and I don't fully understand that reaction... ;-)

Some known ways to chelate excess Iron:

o   Vinegar
o   Fermented foods ^^^
o   Tumeric -- VERY IMPORTANT
o   Phytates (phytic acid...)
o   Tannins (tannic acid...)
o   Yes, Manganese is important, but it, too, needs to be managed by Ceruloplasmin... And food based forms are probably a whole lot better than synthetic supplement forms...

This is VERY MUCH a work in process... I am open to any and all suggestions on how best to address this phenomenon of excess Iron...

Where I think we get into trouble -- me included! -- is making sweeping declarations about "Do this! or Do that!" and NOT take into account the locale of the client, the mineral profile of their soil/water, and other factors that clearly need to be considered....

The practices of Tibetan civilizations vs Peruvian civilizations vs Manhattan civilizations are NOT comparable for a wide variety of reasons. What I am coming to learn is that "mores and standards" are EASILY taken out of context and do not translate well in a completely different climate or setting.

PLEASE STOP THE PRESSES!...

WE NEED TO STOP TALKING ABOUT "LOW IRON!" THIS CONCEPT and TERM MUST BE QUALIFIED...

We run the risk of making the EXACT same mistake that was made for generations re "elevated TSH," thinking that that ONE marker indicated complete Thyroid function. And now we KNOW that, that was ALL WRONG and VERY misleading for millions and millions of folks on this Planet.

There are a series of 8 blood makers that are ESSENTIAL to assess PROPER Iron Metabolism. It is NOT a "one and done!"

http://requestatest.com/mag-zinc-copper-panel-with-iron-panel-testing

We have been trained -- like Circus Bears -- to "be-lie-ve" we were "Iron deficient," when, IN FACT, the majority are SUFFERING from LOW USABLE IRON, AND DROWNING IN EXCESS UNUSABLE IRON...

ALL OF THIS CHAOS BROUGHT TO US BY A LACK OF CERULOPLASMIN (Cp) PRODUCTION FROM OUR LIVERS

THAT ARE OVERLOADED WITH TOXIC LEVELS OF IRON
(that do NOT show on a blood test...).

How "Iron-ic," eh?!?...

Forgive my "yelling ^^^^," but this is an IMPORTANT point and
distinction that ALL need to understand re this VEXING metal!...

The blood can ONLY be made "Red" under the following
conditions:

o   You can NOT make Heme without bioavailable
       Copper...

o   You can NOT make Hemoglobin without bioavailable
       Copper...

o   You can NOT insert the "free, and PROPERLY
       Oxidized Iron" via the Ferrochelatase enzyme without
       bioavailable Copper...

o   You CAN STOP Hypoxia Inducible Factor-1 (HIF-1)
       when there is SUFFICIENT bioavailable Copper...

Do you GET THAT PICTURE?!?...Copper is THE Catalyic Agent
for regulating Iron metabolism.

Forgive me, but my patience is wearing VERY THIN with your
failure to GET THE FULL STORY HERE...

STOP TWISTING THIS INTO AN IRON ISSUE... IT IS NOT AN
IRON ISSUE...

We are led to be-lie-ve that every other person has "Iron
deficiency..."

That is a BOLD FACED LIE... I would suggest that the % that are

TRULY ONLY "Iron deficient" is quite different and much smaller than we are led to think.

THE issue is LOW USABILITY OF THE IRON...

I am seeking to WAKE FOLKS UP that there's WAAAAAAAY MORE to this Iron story and it involves understanding Copper metabolism and the production of THE protein that REGULATES IRON: CERULOPLASMIN...

Recovery START when you changed your focus away from an "Iron ONLY" approach, and take a more wholistic approach?... At least that's how I understand it...

Please know that there is MORE Copper in Liver, than Iron...

That is one reason why the desiccated products work. Iron is the "dummy" and Copper is REALLY running the show...

All is NOT as we've been led to be-lie-ve...

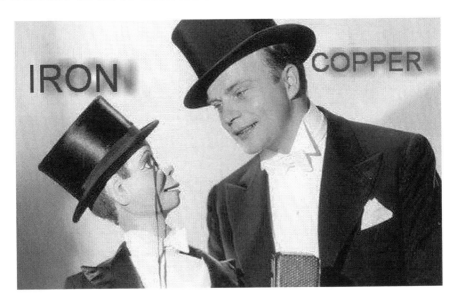

The answer to this vexing Iron-ic issue is NOT to take Copper supplements -- however tempting that may be...

The optimal source for the Copper needed to regulate Iron comes by way of Wholefood Vitamin-C.

There are 20+ steps to increasing the production of Ceruloplasmin. Taking Copper supplements is NOT on it...

Steps To Increase Ceruloplasmin (Cp)

STOP

- STOP Hormone-D ONLY Supplements (KILLS Liver Retinol needed for Cp)
- STOP Calcium Supplements! (Ca BLOCKS Mg & Iron absorption...)
- STOP Iron Supplements! (Fe SHUTS DOWN Cu metabolism...)
- STOP Ascorbic Acid (It disrupts the Copper<>Cp bond)
- STOP HFCS & Synthetic Sugars (HFCS Lowers Liver Copper)
- STOP LOW Fat Diet (Fat is needed for proper Copper absorption)
- STOP Using Industrialized, "Heart Healthy" Oils!
- STOP Using products w/ Fluoride (toothpaste, bottled Water, etc.)
- STOP Taking "Mulit's & Pre-natals" (They have 1st four items ^^^^)

START

- START CLO (1 tsp Rosita's or 1 TBSP Nordic Naturals) for Retinol (Vit-A)
- START Mg supps to lower ACTH & Cortisol (Dose: 5mgs/lb body weight)
- START Wholefood Vit-C (500-800 mgs/day) - source of Copper
- START B7 (Biotin) -- Key for Cu/Fe regulation in Liver
- START B2 (Riboflavin) -- Key for Cu/Fe regulation in Liver
- START Boron -- 1-3 mgs/day (aids in Synthesis of Cp)
- START Taurine to support Copper metabolism in the Liver
- START Ancestral Diet (HIGH Fat & Protein/LOW Carb)
- START Iodine (PREQUISITE: Mg & Se RBC need to be optimal)

Additional Factors to consider regarding Ceruloplasmin:
- Chlorinated water is very hard on Cp production.
- High dose Zinc supplements BLOCK copper absorption.

www.gotmag.org   October 11, 2015

I would venture to say that it was an "Iron dysregulation of your Immune system," that ALLOWED the Bacteria and Parasites associated with Lyme to take root... Superoxide Dismutase plays a VERY powerful role in being the Guard and Bouncer in the body -- WHEN Copper is optimally bioavailable...

That is next to impossible when the body is being flooded with excess, unregulated Iron, because doctors don't take the time to FULLY understand the Iron Metabolism that involves MANY moving parts...

Ideal scenario for an "Iron" Lady:

o Serum Cp = 35
o Serum Fe = ~100
o Serum TIBC = ~285
o Serum Ferritin = 20-50 (per LEADING Cardiologists seeking to STOP Heart events...)

The issue is NOT to "raise" Iron, but make it **MORE bioavailable** by strengthening Cp... Optimize its presence and function -- NOT overwhelm the Liver with Iron supplements. I think that Liver is still a valid and viable way to improve that process...

Please know, Iron is a "dummy" in the body, and Copper/Ceruloplasmin is its MASTER:

http://i1.wp.com/repsonline.org/wpcontent/uploads/2012/07/14EdgarBergenCharlie.jpg

MINERAL FACTOIDS:

1) ALL Tumors must have Iron to survive!...

2) Women with metastasized breast cancer have ELEVATED Ferritin...

Hmmmmmm...

Beware the pursuit of Iron at all costs...

Please know, the issue is NOT Ferritin... The REAL metabolic HERO in Iron Metabolism is your serum level of Ceruloplasmin -- something your Mineral Denialist has NEVER told you about, NOR measured...because they were NEVER trained in this truth.

I believe this is the study that you're looking for:

http://circ.ahajournals.org/content/86/3/803.full.pdf

That's ^^^ a pretty technical article, but here's a wonderful piece by Bill Sardi -- a very gifted health writer -- who will explain why EXCESS IRON AIN'T all it's cracked up to be...

http://knowledgeofhealth.com/revelation-statin-cholesterol-lowering-drugs-work-via-their-ability-to-reduce-Iron-stores-not-cholesterol/

In this article, Sandi highlights the work of Leo R. Zacharski, MD who has discovered the IRON-LOWERING aspect of $tatin$ and advises patients to keep their Ferritin between 20-50 ng/mL. Turns out you'd be better off working with Leeches than $tatin$!!!

And the cherry on the top of this "Iron-ic" issue is this OUTSTANDING article on Iron Fortification that should make EVERYONE in the US, UK, and CANADA quake in their "rusty" boots:

http://freetheanimal.com/2015/06/enrichment-theory-everything.html

Hope that does the trick... There's enough there to make even the most ardent skeptic think twice... And, of course, as you have further questions, please post them!...

Once again, I'm BREAKING with convention to reveal that HIGH Ferritin is NOT a sign of optimal Iron metabolism, despite the chest-beating of Neurologists, Endocrinologist and Thyroid groups.

I'm taking my nod from Cardiologists who are VERY aware of the TOXIC effect of EXCESS Iron -- especially that which is stored in Ferritin...It turns out the Iron in Ferritin, when exposed to Superoxides, is HIGHLY toxic to the cells and the tissues.

At the risk of being PERFECTLY blunt, the Thyroid Groups are clueless about the role of Ferritin in regulating Thyroid function.

At the end of the day, it's ALL about Ceruloplasmin (Cp), and its PROFOUND role to regulate EVERY FACET OF IRON METABOLISM.

Know that Cp contains EIGHT (8) atoms of Copper and IRON DON'T WORK properly without those Copper ions. In effect, Iron is the "Dummy" and Copper is the "Ventroliquist" telling it what to do...

By ALL means, please give up chasing the Iron dummy. But now shift your focus to the Metabolic Mag-ician of the body: Ceruloplasmin!...

I'm a HUGE Christopher Lloyd fan, as well!... And he has perfected that role to a fine art...

This is likely a bit more than you're willing to read, but this is a wonderful overview that sheds important light on the dynamic and damaging relationship Copper and Iron can have with each other, WHEN PRACTITIONERS DON'T HONOR THEIR RESPECIALLYECTIVE ROLES IN THE BODY:

http://www.canaltlabs.com/pictures/site131/content6838/media/The_Copper-Iron_chronicles_The_story_of_an_intimate_relationship.pdf

In my world, Iron is the "Dummy" and Copper is the Ventriloquist/Comedian...(Please forgive my repeated use of this image...I am seeking to overcome your lifelong programming of Iron as the "hero!")

Me thinks it's time for you to upgrade your understanding of the problem:

http://www.ncbi.nlm.nih.gov/pmc/articles/PMC297366/pdf/jcinvest2009-2546.pdf

It is NOT just a Copper issue any more...

To any and ALL still thinking that Mo' Iron is the "best" way to treat Iron Anemia, PLEASE READ the following:

http://www.ncbi.nlm.nih.gov/pmc/articles/PMC297366/pdf/jcinvest 00244-0126.pdf

Please do NOT be fooled by OR be afraid of the "1968" publication date. That is a full twenty years BEFORE BIG Pharma took control of bench medical research...

The stunner is found in the Discussion: "A deficiency of Ceruloplasmin (Cp) is one of the earliest manifestations of Copper deficiency."(Lahey, et al, 1952)

And finally, please know we would be the "Copper deficient swine" in this study...

Hope this clarifies the CRITICAL and CENTRAL role of Copper/Ceruloplasmin in the optimal metabolism of Iron...

Wholefood Vit-C has the Tyrosinase enzyme at the core and inside THAT, are FOUR Copper ions that are key to the production of Ceruloplasmin, which is ESSENTIAL to the proper management of Iron...

It defies ALL Logic, but EVERY facet of Iron metabolism is DEPENDENT upon Copper/Ceruloplasmin. Period!

http://www.ncbi.nlm.nih.gov/m/pubmed/3694287/

Besides the 20% DECREASE in Ceruloplasmin Oxidase Activity -- 2% LOSS would be BAD, by the way... -- It also INTENSIFIES the absorption of Iron...

And while many'll be quick to say, "Isn't THAT a good thing?!?..."

More Iron in a body LOSING Ceruloplasmin Oxidase Activity is VERY DANGEROUS, and is the SOURCE of increased

Oxidative Stress which is the metabolic stimulus is for ALL Chronic Disease...

MAG-pies, please take a moment and re-read what I just said to make sure that what I am stating MAKES SENSE...

For those seeking the TRUTH, please read JUST the last sentence of this Article Abstract:

http://www.ncbi.nlm.nih.gov/pubmed/8907021

*The mineral imbalances in magnesium-deficient rats with dietary iron overload were studied. Forty-four male Wistar rats were divided into six groups and fed six diets, two by three, fully crossed: magnesium adequate or deficient, and iron deficient, adequate, or excess. The concentrations of iron, magnesium, calcium, and phosphorus in tissues of the rats were measured. The results were as follows: (1) The excess iron intake reinforced the iron accumulation in liver and spleen of magnesium deficient rats; (2) The saturation of iron binding capacity was enormously elevated in the magnesium deficient rats fed excess iron; and (3) Dietary iron deprivation diminished the degree of calcium deposition in kidney of magnesium deficient rats. **These results suggest that magnesium-deprived rats have abnormal iron metabolism losing homeostatic regulation of plasma iron, and magnesium deficient rats with dietary iron overload may be used as an experimental hemochromatosis model.**

We would be the "Mg deficient Rats" in this Global experiment with EXCESS "D"ietary Iron!

I rest my case...

May those chasing "LOW Ferritin ONLY" Iron measurements please WAKE UP!!!

Leading Cardiologists are VERY clear about the need to keep Ferritin <50 Mg/dL to AVOID Heart events. And that's a fact. I would trust a Cardiologist 100X BEFORE I would an Endocrinologist!

From what I'm learning, unchecked Iron is THE mechanism for BOTH chronic disease AND constant ca$h flow. Yes, your doctor makes her/his living ONLY when you are $ick...You know that, right?

Harsh comment?... Maybe.
Actual fact?... Absolutely!

When I moved from Chicago (city water with lots of Ca and Mg) and moved to Louisiana (well water with TONS of Iron!) my "Iron-toxic" symptoms went crazy!!! (Hair loss, thyroid dysfunction, passed a Kidney stone -- a 1st for me!!)

I was TOTALLY asleep about Iron 3 years ago!

I am doing EVERYTHING in my power to AWAKEN folks to the "D"anger of excess Iron, ESPECIALLY ITS MAGGIE DEPLETING QUALITIES!...

also know that elevated TIBC = Mg deficiency. The efficiency if transportatinf Iron, via trasnferrin, is gettign enhanced via magnesium...

LOW Ferritin likely means LOW Ceruloplasmin, BUT it MUST be assessed in the CONTEXT of the other Iron markers -- NEVER ALONE! Also, the level of Homosiderin MUST be assessed as that marker reveals the extent to which The Iron in Ferritin is being Oxidized and becoming an agent for INCREASED Free Oxygen Radical Species (ROS)...

ALL IS NOT AS IT SEEMS, NOR AS WE'VE BEEN "TRAINED" TO BELIEVE...

It will take me the rest of 2015 to fully process the MANY stellar studies reviewed on the TOXICITY OF IRON at this excellent website:

http://www.healtheiron.com/iron-infection

Brace yourself! You will not enjoy what this article has to say...

ALL manner of Pathogens: bacterial, fungal, viral, mycotoxin, etc., MUST HAVE IRON TO FLOURISH and GROW....

And where do they find that Iron?!?

Largely from the Iron "stored" in our Ferritin and in our tissues that does NOT show up in blood tests!

A favor, please do the following:

1)   Please take a few minutes and skim these article abstracts. Health-e-Iron has done a masterful job summarizing and highlighting the relevant information...

2)   Please step back and SERIOUSLY re-think your "Allopathetically-inspired Ferritin-loading strategy..."   In my humble opinion, it is RADICALLY flawed and is the source of Iron ESSENTIAL for these Pathogens... (How many on this group have or are actively dealing with Candida, mold, viral issues, etc.?!?...)

3)   Please get a comprehensive blood test that measures ALL facets of Iron, including your Ceruloplasmin (Cp) status.

http://requestatest.com/mag-zinc-copper-panel-with-iron-panel-testing

While this highlighted article is "silent" on Cp's CENTRAL role in Iron management, I believe I've presented compelling evidence and research the past few weeks that should overcome even the greatest of skeptics... Cp makes Copper bioavailable, AND also manages every facet of Iron metabolism via its affect on Iron and the Iron proteins that manage Iron.

And why does MgMan keep obsessing over Iron?!?...

Iron-induced "Oxidative Stress!" INCREASES our MBR (Mg Burn Rate)!

AND...

One of Maggie's greatest gifts is to change the structure of KEY chemicals so that they work optimally inside our bodies and inside our cells. It does this for ATP, and Ceruloplasmin (Cp), and many others! (By the way, there are 3,571 proteins that MUST have Maggie to work properly...)

So, we have come FULL CIRCLE... We have KEEN INSIGHT on how we keep losing our Mg, and we now know that to optimize the function of our Ceruloplasmin, our Mg had best be robust!

Thank you for taking the time to plow through this material. It is NOT an easy read, NOR a pleasant message. But I firmly believe it extends our understanding of the TRUTH of our physiology and and more importantly, the SOURCE of our pathophysiology!

We have MUCH to discuss and MUCH to do to correct our thinking and to correct the notable metal imbalances (low Copper <> high Iron) that are the very ROOT of what ails us...

In my humble opinion, "Ferritin Iron" is akin to "Storage (25OH)-D" AND TSH:

o   Worthless...
o   Completely misleading...
o   Dangerously confusing when NOT in proper CONTEXT
       of the MANY factors needed to assess these confusing
       aspects of our metabolism...

Iron is a PRO-OXIDANT and contributes to ALL facets of Aging...

Francesco S. Facchini, MD referred, very accurately, to Iron as "the aging factor" (Facchini 2002)

There is WAAAAY more Copper than Iron in Liver. Trust me, Thyroid Peroxidase enzyme is "billed" as "Iron dependent," but Iron is the DUMMY in that metabolic Ventriloquist act...

ALL IS NOT AS IT SEEMS!

Wholefood Vit-C that has the enzyme, Tyrosinase, at the core and inside THAT are FOUR Copper atoms making the "Iron Dummy" look good!

Bioavailable Copper is BEST obtained in Wholefood Vit-C -- NOT ASCORBIC ACID!...

Hmmmmm.... Let's see...

Natural wholefood Vitamin-C with bioavailable Copper that is KEY to support the Selenium-dependent process in the Liver to convert T4>>T3

OR...

Synthetic ascorbic palmitate that does WHAT?!?...

It's a quick way to put the spotlight on the truth vs opinion...

Know that as Iron levels rise in tissue -- that do NOT show on blood tests -- that Estrogen levels rise...

Why?!?

In a body LOW in Ceruloplasmin, Cp being a KEY antioxidant, the body must go to its back-up source of Anti-oxidants, especially, Estrogen...

Runaway, stored Iron is likely your culprit...

With some trepidation, I share this:

It appears ALA pulls out Iron (good!) and Copper (not so good...) in its actions of chelation. Caution would be the watchword IF the goal is increased Cp...

Please know, I do NOT profess to understand this "chelation process..." As a rule, I am QUITE leary of it as they act as bulldozers, NOT Cherry pickers...

The Global Social Meme that we are "Iron deficient" is the GREATEST HOAX on this Planet, in my humble opinion...

Iron dysregulation is the PROPER term, and it is an EPIDEMIC worldwide because NO ONE has been told about, NOR trained in the FOUNDATIONAL IMPORTANCE of Ceruloplasmin (Cp), what it does, how to measure it properly, NOR how to increase it naturally...

Iron, without Cp, is a breeding ground for Oxidative Stress!, which is the metabolic trigger for ALL facets of chronic disease. Period!

How Iron-ic is that?!?...

What folks with hemochromatosis need to understand is the status of their Liver's production of Ceruloplasmin (Cp), which is the enzyme that REGULATES every facet of Iron metabolism...

Said another way, the IRPs (Iron Regulatory Proteins) responsible for the absorption, the transport, the metabolic use of (i.e the creation of Hemoglobln), the storage of, and the release from storage of Iron ALL REQUIRE OPTIMAL LEVELS OF Cp...

http://www.ncbi.nlm.nih.gov/pubmed/16831606

It's ALL about understanding how the body REALLY works, NOT how they want us to think it works...

AGAIN, If you have been told that you are "Iron Anemic" and that label was based SOLELY on a Ferritin blood test, I would STRONGLY advise you get this blood test to understand the FULL Monty of your Iron Metabolism:

http://requestatest.com/mag-zinc-copper-panel-with-iron-panel-testing

The SINGLE most important marker for Iron status is to know your Ceruloplasmin (Cp) level, as that is the protein that RUNS the Iron side of the house...

What MOST fail to understand is that Excess, Unmanaged Iron -- due to a LACK OF CERULOPLASMIN (Cp) -- CAUSES *dings* to our DNA... And that SAME protein, Cp, is needed to make Copper bioavailable which is KEY to the function of enzymes (Methyltransferase enzymes, especially) to make genes work properly... They don't turn ON/OFF without these enzymes working properly!

I am HIGHLY skeptical of ANY label that involves the phrase "genetic disorder...", "Gene defect..." OR "mutant!"

But I'm weird that way, because I KNOW how the cellular machinery works and is TOTALLY dependent on mineral activators -- unlike your mis-trained Mineral Denialist...

http://www.ncbi.nlm.nih.gov/pmc/articles/PMC4521784/

Awesome article ^^^^!

It attenuates my ignorance re Curcumin...

The ONLY risk I see is taking a spice with rich, cultural ties and amping it up, which "un-attenuated" Americans and scientists have a penchant for doing...

Ferritin is the LEAST valid marker for TRUE Iron Metabolism status...

If you've been told you're in the "pre-stage" for Cancer, that is PROOF POSITIVE that you have a build-up of Iron in your Breast tissue... THAT MINERAL FACT is a well-kept secret...

http://health-matrix.net/2013/07/06/the-iron-elephant-the-dangers-of-iron-overload/

Why Mg Man has "lost it," and is obsessing over Iron and the PROPER management of Iron:

http://www.ncbi.nlm.nih.gov/m/pubmed/18280258/

Please know, there are 3,571 proteins that REQUIRE Maggie to do their work...

And despite the distorted Iron blood tests and faulty interpretation of Iron status based solely on a Ferritin blood test, please know that we are MAG-nets -- from cradle to grave -- for accumulating Iron each and every day. Key to the optimal management of Iron is Mo' Ceruloplasmin -- NOT Mo' Iron!

Please take a moment, re-read and reflect on that...

Our objective as a community is to reduce our Iron Burden AND preserve our precious stores of life-affirming Magnesium...

The "Set Point" for Iron is established during the weanling period, especially as infants are exposed to TOXIC Iron levels in fortified infant formulas...

And then, as we become adults, THAT is why we ATTRACT Mo' Iron to our Brain...

I realize that the vast majority of folks frequenting my Facebook site are simply looking for "answers" to their ailments. I get that, truly I do, and it's why I spend the MAJORITY of my time interacting with clients -- the world over...

But my passion is to understand HOW & WHY ALL this misery & chronic disease came about, and make sure that I do enough to impart that information & insight onto the "MAG-pies" and "MAG-nets" who grace this august body of healers helping each other...

In my wildest dreams, I never would have imagined three years ago -- yes, it's been 3 "D"og Years of MAG activity for me & the original founders of this mineral-based group of contrarians to convention -- that we would have grown this BIG, nor have tackled SOOOO MANY issues. It's amazing what holding a MIRROR up to "the story" does to reveal the "truth..."

I want folks to better understand why I'm not only gaa-gaa about Maggie, but also a VITAL protein/enzyme produced in our Livers & Brains: Ceruloplasmin (Cp). If the Sun is the "center" of our Universe, I'm coming to regard Cp as the "Sun" of our universe of metabolic activity.

For those that think this is merely "another" protein, you'll find this a fascinating read to better understand the depth and complexity of this protein that has Ferroxidase enzyme activity.

1) Structure & function of Ceruloplasmin:

http://www.ncbi.nlm.nih.gov/pmc/articles/PMC2483498/pdf/d-63-00240.pdf

And what is even more fascinating is to know that Holmberg & Laurell, the discovers of this protein in 1941, identified it to have 8 Copper ions, and that was the case through the 1970's in the literature. And then, suddenly the number of Copper ions dropped to 6-7, and now it's recognized that there are ONLY 6 Copper ions. The re-calibration of the # of Copper ions is hardly due to "superior" diagnostic techniques...

Now anyone who knows me or knows this Group understands the position to STOP the mindless "D"ementia in supplementing

Hormone-D. One of the MAIN reasons is laid out in this article that highlights the VITAL importance of Retinol and Retinoic Acid -- we know this as animal-based Vitamin-A -- in jump-starting the production of Cp. Given that Vit-A & Hormone-D are biological antagonists, it's impossible to do so when "D"rowning our Liver in that vogue supplement that is wildly myth-understood...

2) Importance of Retinol in producing Ceruloplasmin:

http://jn.nutrition.org/content/117/9/1615.long

It's well chronicled in the literature that Ceruloplasmin (Cp) is the biological agent to keep Iron in a proper valence (# of electrons), and mostly importantly, keep it moving in & around the cell. The scientists like to refer to it as "cellular Iron efflux," but that's a fancy way of saying "keep it moving!"

That's the IDEAL state for Iron... It is NOT meant to be "STORED" and measuring Iron in its storage state -- via the Ferritin molecule -- makes NO sense at all. It's akin to selecting a car based SOLELY on the size of the Trunk, and IGNORING the size & efficiency of the engine, AS WELL AS the overall handling of the car... (Who does THAT make sense to?!?...Selecting a car based on its Trunk?...)

And what's also known is that Ceruloplasmin (Cp) elevates in response to Inflammation. This is a biological certainty that has been encoded going back millennia of millennia... And now, BIG Pharma is seeking to apply the same MYTH-information strategy re Cp that kept us kidnapped for 60 yrs re Cholesterol. They want us to see Cp as the BAD guy, and do what we can to "lower" it...

Which makes absolutely NO sense, but its elevation is consistent, particularly during an Inflammatory state.

And what they are forgetting to tell us is that Ceruloplasmin must be folded properly and have optimal amino acid composition to

FUNCTION FULLY as an Enzyme... And the enzyme of choice is Ferroxidase, which is the active component of Cp that REGULATES Iron status and Iron movement...

And this was MOST confusing until I came across pearl yesterday and learned WHY Iron has to be in a certain valence to TURN OFF the activity of a KEY enzyme that used by neutrophils to KILL bacteria.

3) Ferric Iron (Fe++) Inactivation of Myeloperoxidase (MPO):

http://www.jbc.org/content/234/9/2486.full.pdf

What has also become clear is that "Inflammation" is actually an immune response to an "infection," but WITHOUT the Pathogen!! You might want to re-read that sentence again, slooooooowly, to understand what "Inflammation" is... (It's also important to know that LACK of sufficient Magnesium is the cellular state that TRIGGERS the Inflammatory Cascade...)

And then the universe dropped this pearl into my lap -

4) Cp is an Endogenous Inhibitor of Myeloperoxidase (MPO):

http://www.jbc.org/content/288/9/6465.full

So, once again, Ceruloplasmin comes to the rescue to regulate, or modulate the MPO response. That is HUGE, and it makes sense that biologically it's coming to the scene of the crime, whether it's got the enzyme capacity or not. It's almost like "muscle memory" only this is "immune memory..." And what Cp is doing is MANAGING the Iron to stay in the right state and stay active...

Now, for those seeking to understand WHY there's always a death or two at a Marathon (Rick Malter, PhD...) this puts an entirely different spin on it. Endurance exercise DEPLETES our

119

minerals, especially Maggie, and that sets the stage for an Inflammatory response in our heart, which then triggers a RISE of MPO, and if were SHORT on Ceruloplasmin, the degradation of Heme releases Mo' Iron, which accelerates Lipid Peroxidation (we know that as "Plaque"...) and it's good night, Irene for that Cp-deficient runner. And know that chronic "Stress!" is a MAJOR cause of under-production of Cp in the Liver...

5) MPO is elevated following a Marathon, endurance exercise:

http://ajcp.oxfordjournals.org/content/126/6/888

6) MPO >> HOCl- >> Heme Degradation >> Iron Release...

http://www.plosone.org/article/fetchObject.action...

OK, so this has to be among the MOST boring and "academic" Posts, not just on MAG, but on all of FB, wouldn't you agree?!?...

Well, here's the punch line...

One of my colleagues/clients/fellow Iron researcher/friends, Maria Dolores Chagas Oliveira, has helped me see the light re HOW Ceruloplasmin is getting tweaked, and losing its Ferroxidase function. It is the being CAUSED by the "nitration of a key amino acid, Tyrosine." Be careful, this is NOT for the faint of heart or anyone looking for a quick read:

7) Nitric Oxide, Oxidants and Protein Tyrosine Nitration:

http://www.pnas.org/content/101/12/4003.full.pdf

And what's the BEST way to "Nitrate Tyrosine?!?"

Expose it to Superoxide radicals and NO2 that is CAUSED by excess, unmanaged Iron. This idea that we are "Iron deficient" is beyond ridiculous, despite the countless articles that say we are. Imho, it is absolutely just the OPPOSITE!

So, we've come FULL circle. Iron is THE "Stressor!" that is CAUSING excess loss of Maggie, and now we come to realize that it is the CAUSATIVE agent to create Oxygen Stress, AND Nitrogen Stress that is at the heart of neutering Ceruloplasmin, the very protein/enzyme that is ESSENTIAL to properly manage this toxic metal...

How Iron-ic is that?!?...

God bless you all... Hope you find this Post helpful and informative... Come 2016, we will be focusing more & more on how to correct this metabolic imbalance that pervades the universe...

MERCURY: FACTORS TO CONSIDER

My working hypothesis is that Mercury has ALWAYS been toxic.

What is different today is a decidedly LOWER level of Bioavailable Copper that is especially effective at neutralizing Oxidative Stress, via its direct production/activation of CuZnSOD and indirect activation of Catalase (Iron ain't nothing without bioavailable Copper...), and Glutathione (GSH Px is Copper dependent...)

Why is Copper sucking wind these days?...

o   Relentless levels of "Stress!" in a society DEPRIVED of minerals...

o   HFCS that CAUSES LOW levels of Liver Copper AND HIGH Levels of Liver Iron, which destroys Copper metabolism...

o   Glyphosate Toxicity (RoundUp!) that targets the chelation of key minerals, especially Copper and Maggie...

o   Blind supplementation of Hormone-D that destroys Liver Vit-A (retitol, animal based) that is KEY to the production of Ceruloplasmin (Cp)...

o   Blind supplementation of Ascorbic Acid that causes the Copper ions to be "ripped off" the Ceruloplasmin, thereby causing a loss of oxidase enzyme function...

I'm deeply suspicious that in 1982 the design of Mercury amalgams changed by putting MORE Copper in it, which INCREASED Hg's toxicity 20X... per Anne Ann Louise Gittleman...

That is NOT an accident... When did Glyphosate and HFCS come on the scene?... about the SAME time... Almost like it was planned...

Now we're dealing with a generation of Methyltransferase enzyme failures, aka MTHFR... And what mineral activates the Methyltransferase family of enzymes?... Copper!

What's the KEY agitator in "D"estroying THAT dynamic?...

Mercury!

Forgive me... I SMELL A RAT...

Mercury has been on this Planet for a LOOOOOONG time...

Mercury has been used in dental products since the 1860's...

Mercury Toxicity seems to have GROWN in impact just within the last generation...

Is the inverse ever possible, i.e. that LOW bioavailable Copper <> coupled with HIGH Iron Overload sets the stage for us to BECOME **more** prone to Mercury Toxicity?...

When LOW bioavailable Cu/HIGH unusable Iron -- BOTH due to a lack of optimal Ceruloplasmin -- exist, the body's ability to make Anti-Oxidant Enzymes is compromised, as they are ALL directly or indirectly dependent on Copper to make (SOD, CAT, GSH)...

I'm just curious about the Chicken/Egg dimension of this ubiquitous Mercury condition that seems to have gotten WORSE when:

o   Copper was added to Mercury amalgams in 1982 making then 20X more toxic...

o   HFCS got added MAJORLY (early 1980's) to our diet and has KNOWN properties of LOWERING Liver Copper and RAISING Liver Iron...

o   Prevalence of Glyphosate (early 1980's) that has KNOWN properties of LOWERING Liver Copper and RAISING Liver Iron...

o   The adjuvant for Vaccines was changed (early 1980's) from just Mercury to Aluminum... Hmmm... Turns out two issues at play:

   1)   Aluminum whips up Iron in the body...

   2)   They STILL wash the ingredients in Thimerisol, and the Mercury content is even GREATER now than before...

Please know, I'm NOT a Luddite on this Mercury issue...

I'm beginning to wonder to what extent it is FOSTERED by the imbalance of our mineral soil, aka as our gut and Liver, and our innate inability to detoxify this heavy metal?!?...

Two KEY numbers to know BEFORE pursuing Amalgam removal:

o   How many times has this dentist removed amalgams?...

o How many patients have you personally talked to see how good they felt FOLLOWING this procedure?...

I would contend you DO have options...

I would strongly recommend you read this book BEFORE you have your procedure done:

Hal Huggins, "It's ALL in Your Head"

URL: http://www.amazon.com/Its-All-Your-Head-Amalgams/dp/0895295504

If your dentist is NOT Huggins certified and hasn't extensive experience, it simply is NOT worth the risk of doing this dental procedure. Please know, among my SICKEST clients are ALL folks who can trace their "D"ownturn to a "D"ental procedure, especially Amalgam removal...

MINERALS: FACTS TO CONSIDER

Folks...

Mineral levels and ratios...

Drive Enzyme function...

Many of which are MADE by Endocrine Glands...

Minerals FIRST...

It's basic, it's boring, but it's BIOLOGICAL...

o   Organic foods...
o   Spring water that's UN-touched by human hands...
o   Anderson's Mineral drops...
o   Anderson's Fortisalt...
o   Aussie Minerals...
o   Sea Salt...
o   REAL Pepper...
o   Spices...
o   Herbs...
o   AND Seaweed!

POTASSIUM: FACTORS TO CONSIDER

Especially the ease with which we can ask or make compelling comments on FB, the mastery of mineral metabolism dictates measurement and assessment of the OVERALL mineral profile to better understand the contexts for your reactions to this process.

Indeed, we are ALL different -- both OUTSIDE and INSIDE. And that difference needs to be illuminated to the best know how to correct the mineral imbalances and ratios...

Know that if your Potassium is rising in the Serum that is a "Stress!" reaction... Potassium belongs INSIDE the cell, and ONLY comes out when provoked...

Magnesium guards Potassium status at the cell wall by regulating the Na/K-ATPase pump that keeps most Na OUTSIDE the cell and most K INSIDE the cell...

Under "Stress!", we lose Magnesium... it's how we're wired as a species...

When Potassium levels are changing it's KEY to look for what's happening to Magnesium... Mg loss PRECEDES Potassium loss, AND Magnesium repletion PRECEDES Potassium repletion...

This has been WELL established in the research over the last 80+ years...

The fact that your mineral denialist doctor NEVER assesses Mg status when looking at Potassium status should send a *chill* down EVERYONE'S spine...

Okay.. Let me see if I understood this right.. Stress causes Magnesium to deplete... which in turn causes potassium to deplete. So, that causes K to get released from the cells into the blood… so higher levels of K in serum tests are indicative of stress and Mg depletion??

Yes!, you, da man!...

And now that you're Dad's drinking the Cool-Aid, here's the graduate level course on Maggie, in a stuffy NEPHROLOGY journal, no less:

http://ckj.oxfordjournals.org/content/5/Suppl_1.toc

It's a BIG deal to devote an ENTIRE Journal to ONE Mineral!...

What I've learned since 2009, is that what causes low Potassium, is typically one of the following...

o   Blood Pressure Medication (Diuretics, especially)
o   B12 Supplements
o   Vitamin-D ONLY Supplements
o   Excess unbound Copper and/Iron

Find the cause and seek to restore and rebalance....

Low Potassium will cause "MAG"nesium loss.

You need Potassium to break down sugars!!

Vitamin-A (Retinol) is your primer for Potassium in the body...

SALT: FACTORS TO CONSIDER

We use 5-7 different forms:

o   Celtic Sea Salt..
o   Redmonds Real Salt
o   Hawaiian pink salt...
o   Anderson's Forti-salt (this stuff is amazing!)
o   Black Salt...
o   Paprika (high in Vit-C)
o   many other spices/herbs depending on the dish...

Val Anderson: the company that I work with makes FortiSalt, which gives you a full salty flavor with less than half the sodium of table salt and provides a higher % RDA/DV of magnesium and every essential trace element (excluding iron) than it does of sodium. It also has more potassium per serving than a potassium supplement. It tastes like salt but richer and more complex and has won chef's awards like the iTQi Superior Taste Award. www.utmin.com

Please know folks, I have no formal, or informal ties to Val's company...

I simply value his mineral genius (he used to hang with the great Mildred S. Seelig, MD of Magnesium fame and others...) and his family's mineral products are among the BEST on this Planet...

Simply a random act of kindness for a guy and a company that has our back... I'm most grateful!

SILVER: FACTORS TO CONSIDER

Silver (Ag) brings short-term relief, AND long-term devastation to Copper status... Ag sits BELOW Cu on the Periodic Table and knocks it out, which is NOT a good solution, over the long haul...

All I know is that as you study the Periodic Table, you'll note that Silver sits directly below Copper and Cadmium sits directly below Zinc. It is a known fact that Cadmium (typically found in cigarette smoke) displaces Zinc, and what appears to be true is that Silver displaces its neighbor to the North...(Ie. Copper...)

The Bactericidal properties of Copper are legendary, but Silver has become a popular form of "natural anti-biotic", but its properties are not without impact to the innate immune function that depends on optimal levels of bioavailable Copper...

I would NOT use Silver... I would work to strengthen the bioavailability of your Copper...

Please know, minerals are not pieces on a game board... They are not interchangeable as you suggest...

Last licks, it's important to remember that MTHR NATURE preferred anti-biotics in humans is Cu,Zn-SOD. When Copper levels are optimal, this KEY enzyme is a powerhouse neutralizing pathogens and the free radicals.

VITAMINS

B-VITAMINS

It is worth noting that in the 1930's scientists studied the effect of taking Copper out of B5 and note that it CAUSED Black rats to turn White...

Hmmmm...

It's ALSO worth noting that Merck was awarded a patent in 1947 to create the synthetic form of B5 => Calcium D-Pentothenate... You will note this form is now found on <u>ALL</u> Bottled B's -- all over the world...

Is it B5 that we need or the Copper ion(s) that might be needed to address this metabolic process...

It is further worth noting that Ferrochelatase enzyme is ENTIRELY Copper dependent and is the rate-limiting step to make Heme....

Hmmmmm...

I know I'm a total bore, but it's biological...

Homo Normalus RUNS on Minerals, especially Mg and Copper.

Period!...

What mineral(s) are in that synthetic form of B5?...

MTHR NATURE has tons of Copper in these CLASSIC forms of B-Vitamins:

o   Bee Pollen and Bee products...

o   Nutritional Yeast....

o   Rice Bran...

o   Organ meats, especially Liver, Kidney, Heart etc...

Bottled B's are lacking the catalytic agent, Copper, in my humble opinion... They are designed to stimulate, NOT rebuild.

It AIN'T the Vitamin... it's the PRECIOUS Cargo that they deliver that is SOOOO important to the Enzyme function...
And now MY head is spinning!...

Ethanol BLOCKS biosynthesis of Acetyl CoA...

Hmmmm...

Has anyone checked the MOST ubiquitous form of Ethanol in our diet today is HFCS...

Also, it's intriguing that they say Cupric (2+) Copper affects this process, but are SILENT on Cuprous (1+) Copper... I'd bet the farm that bioavailable Copper -- i.e. Cu(1+) – is absolutely KEY to a successful biosynthetic process...

And this is the dysfunctional process being undertaken ALL OVER OUR BODY because it's "What We Eat, Eats" that REALLY Matters, and feeding Pigs Cu(2+)SO4 for growth -- PREVENTS ours!...

I am increasingly skeptical of what "Bottled B's" are REALLY delivering...

I'm moving away from "B"ottled B's... they are TOO synthetic and LACK the Copper that is key to making ALL these "B"lessed vitamins work!...

In that second set of ten factors outlining the elements that have been SPECIFICALLY identified in the Research as being

ESSENTIAL to the production of Cp...

So, "D"itch those Bottled B's... and turn your attention to those delivered by MTHR NATURE:

o   Bee Pollen: 1/2 tsp/day...

o   Nutritional Yeast OR Rice Bran: 1-2 Tbsp/day...

o   Beef Liver: 1oz/week (a piece the size of your palm)

Yummmmmmm...

MUCH "B"etter for you, too!

I've NOT researched this, YET, but someone noted the other day that activated vitamin-B6, P5P -- which is ENTIRELY synthetic -- has a potential "D"ownside of binding up Copper... Now if that's true, which I'm a bit confused and conflicted over, your body would revolt over any agent that would lower your already LOW levels of Copper...

Please know that MOST who "think" they have B12 deficiency, in fact, have a LACK of bioavailable Copper...Copper plays a very quiet, but important role in these vitamins....

All is NOT as it seems...

CHLOROPHYLL

Chlorophyll is the source of plant life! We regularly use Standard Process Chlorophyll Capsules as a therapeutic agent...

As for "containing Copper" -- that is a synthetic compound that has REMOVED Mg and inserted Copper.

http://nullo.com/chlorophyllin.html

The fact that "Chlorophyllin" has been "approved" by the FDA should clue you in on its "safety!"

Chlorophyll -- YES!
Chlorophyllin -- NO!

It is also intriguing to reflect on the identical nature of the chemical structure of Chlorophyll (plants) and Hemoglobin (animals). What makes them different:

o   Chlorophyll has Mag at the centre....
o   Hemoglobin has Fe at the centre...

It's also intriguing to reflect on the biological and physiological antagonism of Mg<>Fe in our own bodies....

COD LIVER OIL

I am trying to educate us all to the "D"ark side of the Lipid Industry... I've known for a decade or more that the oils that we've been TRAINED to use -- the "Heart Healthy" Oils -- are ANYTHING but...

What I am learning -- painfully... -- is that this dynamic extends to the world of CLO, as well...

Am I frustrated?... Totally!....

Do we have reason to be cautious?... Certainly!....

Will we stay vigilant and choose wisely?... Absolutely!...

And for anyone who has verifiable, independent information that challenges what I am is saying, by all means, please bring it to our attention...

We're ALL frustrated by the outright "D"eception and "D"isinformation that PERVADES the food and supplement industry...

Here's an IMPORTANT flow chart to understand the industrial process for Margarine that MOST people eat without giving consideration how it is really made:

http://mobile.dudamobile.com/site/preventdisease?url=http%253A%252F%252Fpreventdisease.com%252Fnews%252F14%252F041514_Do-People-That-Eat-Margarine-Know-How-Its-Manufactured.shtml

if you think this is irrelevant, good luck finding REAL butter the

next time you eat out or go to buy it at the grocery store. Margarine is now~90+% of the options, in a typical grocery store... And why is Butter SOOO important?
It has ALL the Fat Soluble Vitamins: A/D/E/K, unlike Olive Oil and Coconut Oil! (Did you ever check that, in a Nutrient Data Table?!?...)

So, it looks like another recommended source of Vit-A and D may be biting the dust... I do agree, I wish we could hear from Nordic Naturals directly. But I also have confidence in the research and position that is provided.

We need to remain vigilant and open-minded. These are challenging times to move safely through the supplement industry, that appears to be seeking to waste our $€£¥ and bankrupt our health...

I, for one, am quite "D"isgusted by the whole lot!...

Many, many folks have been "D"uped by the belief that they are Vit-"D"eficient, when in fact that is just ANOTHER nutritional scam to add to the litany of "D"ietary scams that our intellect and sanity have been abused by for the last 60+ years...

Hormone-D, it's NOT a vitamin, has a decided ability to BURN OUT the Retinol, (animal-based Vit-A), in the Liver, which is a vital component of our metabolism... REAL Cod Liver Oil, the way MTHR NATURE intended it, has ~10X more Vit-A to Hormone-D to keep things in balance in these halcyon days of "extremist nutrition!"...

When folks take 5,000 IUs of Hormone-D, they SHOULD ALSO be taking ~50,000 IUs of Retinol... It is a VERY RARE practitioner or article that EVER advises that nutritional foundation...

CLO (Cod Liver Oil), when properly extracted and bottled, , is a great source of this BALANCED SOURCE of two key Fat Soluble Nutrience: Vitamin-A and Hormone-D...

Do I personally "use" CLO?...

Here's how I make/intake Hormone-D:

o   I live in Louisiana where there's more sunshine in a week than I saw in a month in Chicago... I walk regularly to soak up the rays!

o   I eat two farm-fresh eggs from girls that are allowed to eat bugs and grasses, etc. OUTSIDE... Think of chickens as little solar panels...

o   I eat a high-end bacon each day from pigs that graze outside too... Pigs are bigger solar panels...

o   I eat dairy products from cows that graze on REAL grass OUTSIDE... Cows are even bigger solar panels... And yes, these animals INFUSE the goodness of the Sun into their products...

o   I eat fish on occasion, but not regularly, especially sardines and other small, oily fish in salads...

o   I take Standard Process Cod Liver Oil on a rare occasion, but know that I fully intend to research its source, and HOW it's processed...

I have NEVER taken Hormone-D as a supplement. It never made sense to me... Thank Heavens!...

As for healthy, I'm better than most, but in light of my ancestry, a far cry from "ideal"...

o   Mom: High BP, Colitis (Colostomy for 18 months), 1 stroke, 3 heart attacks, HEAVY drinker, lifelong smoker (started age 12) but despite ALL that, she was a GREAT Mom!... She passed away on the night before her 67th B-day...

o   Dad: Schizophrenic, and Manic Depressive. Died of Lung Cancer a couple of weeks before his 55th B-day...

o   Maternal Grandmother: Kidney Disease (1/2 of 1 kidney at the end), 3 heart attacks, breast cancer, heavy drinker, cataracts, high blood pressure, etc. Died when she was in her mid-70's...

o   Paternal Grandmother: had a nervous breakdown and spent last 25 years of her life in a mental hospital... it's speculated that she had Alzheimer's Disease...

o   Older sister: Breast Cancer (2x), High blood pressure, Lupus, Diabetes, rheumatoid arthritis, weight issues, etc.

I share all that with you to create a better "context..." I made different choices in my life. There was NO end of "Stressors!" but I decided I would NOT smoke, NOT drink in excess, that i would eat REAL food (Eat for Your Blood Type and Atkins SAVED my derriere), NOT fall for Margarine, etc., NOT fall for booga-wooga Cholesterol, NOT take Doctors too seriously, and NOT allow the demons from my early upbringing were always trying to take hold of me...

I have long connected with the saying:
"Destiny is a matter of choice, not a matter of chance..."

I am hardly a paragon of health... but I'm waaaaay ahead of many that are in their early 60's... And as I look over my family's litany of illnesses, I can safely say they are ALL born of "Stress!"-induced mineral loss... especially Mg and Copper dysregulation...

What I am NOW coming to realize is the role "Iron-Stress" has played in their lives and poor health.

I truly believe that Nordic Naturals - Artic is still a good and valid product. But it's not "perfect!" (What product is?...) There are many members of MAG that are getting positive results with Nordic... I think it's fine to use this product, but know that there is ALWAYS a better product, whether we're talking CLO, B-Vitamins, Minerals, or whatever...

We simply need to know that information is very carefully constructed on products... It requires discernment and a willing to consider all aspects of whatever we're working with in our diet and protocols...

The BIGGEST issue today is that FAAAAAAAR TOOOOO MANY people are "D"rowning is a certain supplement and NOT MANY folks are aware of the "D"ownside of this nutritional SCAM. The reason for pursuing CLO, is NOT to address this mythical need for "D," but to offer up a NATURAL and BALANCED (how that's for an idea, eh?...) food that has been used for hundreds (thousands?) of years...

The HIDDEN issue for MANY folks is that their Ceruloplasmin (Cp) function is very much challenged by the over consumption of this "D"amaging "D"aily "D"ietary "D"ictum...

If we take a strict stance on HTMAs, however, it is not always recommended that a "Slow" Oxidizer be taking Hormone-D, and the slow oxidizers pattern accounts for ~80% of all HTMAs. But the reason why we're pursuing tCLO in this case is to offset the GROSS IMBALANCE of Vit-A:D, and underproduction of Cp that clearly exists by SOOOOO MANY having anemic Potassium in addition, we are using as natural a form of CLO as is possible to correct this "D"ysfunction...

It is a balancing act...

Totally agree!

CLO has notable levels of Retinol (animal-based Vit-A) Know that there are are two ESSENTIAL precursors to make Ceruloplasmin (Cp):

o   Bio-available Copper (typically in Wholefood Vitamin C)
o   13-cis Retinoic Acid (derived from Retinol)

Also, each Cp molecule contains 8 atoms of Copper...

Ascorbic Acid destroys the bond between, Cp and Copper and STOPS Cp's ability to use the Ferroxidase enzyme and thus Iron a USABLE element inside our body...

Get your Copper from REAL wholefood Vit-C...

Get your 13-cis Retinoic Acid from CLO...

Green Pastures is very popular, but they haven't published data on their ratio of Vit-A:Vit-D for THREE (3) years! TILT! Also Kaayla Daniels, PhD, has pulled back the curtain on this product to reveal much that should cause pause...

They are in a parking lot pending their willingness to reveal what they are selling.. Rosita's and Nordic Naturals Artic (NOT Artic-D) are willing to state openly their content of nutrients..

CAVEAT EATOR, especially when it comes to CLO!

Please RETURN the Green Pastures and USE the ones recommended: Rosita's or Nordic Naturals...

Do NOT use the Green Pastures "because you bought it, so I'll use it up..." I've had MORE clients use that strategy to dig their holes "D"EEPER... It is an ill-fated pursuit that has proven itself with scores and scores of clients, who suffered mightily, holding onto supplements that they should have swiftly shed...

VITAMIN D: "D"ISTRESSING

BEFORE we start on the Vit-D issue, know that the Liver LIVES on Retinol (animal based vitamin-A). And the MORE synthetic, hormone-D it's exposed to, the LESS VIABLE the Retinol is, which then means that Iron regulation is affected, because Ceruloplasmin (Cp) production is triggered by 13-cis retinoic acid, a derivative of Retinol.

To fully understand Hormone-D, you need to know the following:

o   Mag RBC

o   Storage Hormone-D (25(OH)D)

o   Active Hormone-D (1,25(OH)D2)

o   Ionized Calcium

o   Potassium RBC (excess Calcium CAUSES Renal Potassium Wasting)

NOW let's jump.....
This article is likely to "D"istress even the most ardent fan of Hormone-D:

http://www.ncbi.nlm.nih.gov/pmc/articles/PMC1866639/pdf/1732.pdf

I plan to write a longer blog about this research and its implications, but please know these three key issues: (There are 6 summary points at the end of the article that are worth carefully reviewing...)

143

o   Calcium rushing INTO the cell is NOT good! This implies
         that Maggie is rushing OUT!... (That is called a CLASSIC
         "Stress!" response!...)

o   Loss of ATP is NEVER a good development for the cell!...
         The state of Dis-ease ALWAYS follows the LOSS of
         energy (spelled Mg-ATP inside the cell)... And what is tied
         to a loss of energy?... Mg drops OFF the ATP molecule
         when the pH of the cell drops below 6.2! Without yhe
         steroe chemical role of Mg, the cell can no longer
         recognise "ATP!"

Hmmmmmmm...

o   Having unbound Iron cavorting in the cell is NEVER a
         good idea due to its profound ability to GENERATE free
         radicals, aka, Reduced Oxygen Species (ROS) -- these
         are the VERY ORIGIN OF THE AGING PROCESS...

And how does Iron BECOME "unbound?"... Increased levels of
Hormone-D overwhelm the Retinol, (animal-based Vit-A), in the
Liver, which is a CRITICAL precursor to making Ceruloplasmin
(Cp), which is an ESSENTIAL protein needed to prevent Iron
(and Copper...) from becoming Oxidizing fiends in the cell...

A vital issue to know: **Cp is, in fact, an anti-oxidant!**

What is NOTABLY absent from this study is ANY mention of
either Magnesium or Copper... And in case you didn't know this,
it is physiologically IMPOSSIBLE to talk about Calcium, without
assessing Maggie, and the same can be said for Iron vs
Copper...

This gap in the breadth of this study is just further proof of the century-long censorship of the KEY minerals that RUN THE BODY...

For those that take the time to actually read this study, it should send a *chill* down your spine...

After my read of this article for the third time, I checked in with my mentor, Rick Malter, PhD, to make sure I was "reading this correctly..." He, too, was quite stunned by the scope of this study and its implications...

Hormone-D "KILLS" Retinol, which is the critical precursor to making Cp in the Liver... It's been the STEALTH agent for Copper and Iron dysregulation for the last decade...

Much to EVERYONE'S lack of awareness...

But the point of my post is to enlighten folks re the impact of D-only supplementation -- it "D"evastates Mg status! And numerous OTHER minerals as noted in the study...

THAT, after all, is the purpose of MAG... I am NOT here to correct FALSE and "D"eceptive blood tests of Storage-D...

Please know, I am STUNNED -- daily -- by folks' obsession, worldwide, to address their "D"eficiency without a complete understanding of its impact on their Mg metabolism, nor any awareness that it is affectively BOTH their Copper and Iron metabolism...

THAT is the purpose of this article... to CHALLENGE the "D"earth of understanding about what Calcitirol REALLY "D"oes INSIDE the body, and INSIDE the cells...

I trust you'll understand my moving beyond these questions...

Based on WHAT testing did your Mineral Denialist reach the conclusion that you needed Mo' Calcium?...

Please read:

http://www.mgwater.com/gacontro.shtml

http://www.naturalnews.com/038286_magnesium_deficiency

Regrettably, your practitioner's got it Affagato (that's Italian for "backwards!")

For those that take Calcium and D supplements, when was the last time that you assessed your overall mineral status via an HTMA and targeted Vit-D blood tests (Active-D AND Storage-D) to determine what is REALLY going on?... MANY MAG-pies and their doctors have been quite surprised to see what the 1,25(OH) -- Active-D-- reveals about the "D"ynamics that are ACTUALLY taking place...

Don't think I'm "pimping" for Mo' Business... that is the farthest thing from my mind...

I'm very concerned that people read articles and/or take the advice of their equally ill-informed neighbors, or worse yet, their undertrained doctors, to consume this calcium mineral that turns the body to stone!...

Please, take a moment, and some time, to do your due diligence on your own body -- with proper testing -- that you will NOT find in your Mineral Denialist's office...

Many folks that I work with present with what on the surface appears to be a "chaotic gaggle of symptoms" -- at least that's how they've been "trained" -- like Circus Bears -- to see it...

What I set out to do, in the process of the consult, is create a context for how chronic "Stressors!" have set the stage for Mg loss, which then sets the stage for the complete dysregulation of Copper and Copper-dependent enzymes, given that the assault of ACTH and Cortisol (which RISE as Mg levels FALL...) affects the Liver's production of this KEY Cu protein, called Ceruploplasmin...And when its off, so too, is metabolism...

And what then transpires from this discussion is the realization that there's a finely ordered "Solar system" -- complete with rotating Planets (symptoms) -- revolving around a "Sun" that is, for a fact, LACK OF BIO-AVAILABLE Copper... in large part due to a lack of optimal levels of Ceruloplasmin (Cp) being made in the Liver for a whole host of reasons...

This, of course, is NOT the entirety of the situation, but only ~90% of it...

To what extent can the Obsession over Hormone-D affect the status and function of Retinoic Acid:

http://www.sciencedirect.com/science/article/pii/S088875431100 1583

We will NOT change this dysfunctional medical/pharmaceutical system...

We WILL change the # of people who believe in it and are willing to RISK THEIR LIVES with it...

A General CHOOSES his/her battle... and that's MINE!...

147

Here's the "D"eal, folks...

There is a MAJOR "D"ifference between "The STORY" and "The TRUTH"...

Most of what we read on the internet is "The Story," that we are expected to "believe" in AND "act on...

"It is the "Social Construction of Reality!"

It is NOT the Truth...

Classic examples from a nutritional standpoint include:

o   **Cholesterol is "D"emonic and will kill you**... OMg! (Cardiologists and waiting rooms full of terrified patients actually believe that...)

o   **Calcium builds strong bones**.. OMg! (People have been poisoned for decades with excess Calcium because Mineral Denialists have NO CLUE how Bone Matrix is built around 18 nutrients and that Calcium is the "D"umb Front Lineman of the lot... By the way, Hormone-D is "Calcium" ON STEROIDS!...)

o   **Iron-poor blood/anemia is CAUSED by too little Iron...** OMg! (MAG me with a spoon... ALL Iron proteins are Copper-dependent, which was established in the 1860's... NO, that is NOT a typo!!!)

So, regrettably, the (M)asses (~98%) prefer to NOT rock the boat, choose to "believe" The Story, and choose to SUFFER mightily from their "D"ementia...

Remember, "D"estiny is a matter of choice, NOT a matter of chance...

The rest of us, ~2% of the population is willingly craving, and seeking The TRUTH... And that's what MAG is ALL about...

Please know that 99.9% of ALL documents on Google Scholar are paid for and presented by BIG Pharma... Unless you know the "code" of how they are contructed and crafted, you will NOT know the TRUTH of these "D"elightful and "D"eceitful research studies...

Yes, I am a Conspiracist, except it's NO LONGER a Conspiracy when you can PROVE IT, right?... ;-)

All I can say is that there is TRUE INTENT is getting folks to "D"rown in Hormone-D. It is the MOST over-rated and mis-understood nutritional miscreant in the ENTIRE fields of health nutrition...

And if you elect to believe that blah, blah, blah, I've got BOTH a used-BMW and a Bridge that I'd like to sell ya!...

Please know, I find it most "D"isarming when ostensibly smart folks are sooooo easily "D"ecieved... I thought the credo for Harvard was "VERITAS"... Has that changed, too?...

Please read: www.ncbi.nlm.nih.gov/pubmed

http://www.ncbi.nlm.nih.gov/pmc/articles/PMC3915480/?report=printable

Let me put it this way... 99.9% of the non-scholar folks who read articles on Google Scholar are NOT savvy enough to know FACT from FICTION... I know I wasn't when I started out 7 years ago...

But now with ~2,500 articles under my belt, I can very quickly assess the BS factor in those studies and determine the gist of the study and the extent to which they HONOR or DEFAME the natural metabolism of the human body...

It is NOT in print -- that much is for sure!...It is often implied by what they FAIL to say....

I think THIS is faaaar more important and telling about the untold "D"ark Side to the alleged "Sunshine" Hormone:

http://www.ncbi.nlm.nih.gov/m/pubmed/24204002/

People are CLUELESS about the "D"ysregulation and "D"ysfunction they are "D"irecting by their "D"aily "D"rowning in this toxin!

http://www.westonaprice.org/wp-content/uploads/2013/07/fall2012masterjohnfig5.jpg

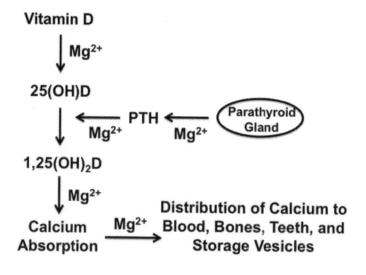

You might study this person's experience carefully:
http://www.growyouthful.com/comment-ailment-remedy.php?ailmentNo=347&remedyNo=3

Do you know your Mag RBC?...
Do you know your 1,25(OH) Active Hormone-D level?...
Do you know your Potassium level?...

I would use Magnesium Oil 100X to SOLVE this obvious nutritional deficiency BEFORE ever allowing synthetic, Soy-based Hormone-D to ever touch my lips...

As for the Hormone-D, please know that the Liver LIVES on Retinol. And the MORE synthetic, hormone-D it's exposed to, the LESS VIABLE the Retinol (animal-based Vitamin-A) is, which then means that Iron regulation is affected, because Ceruloplasmin (Cp) production is triggered by 13-cis retinoic acid, a derivative of Retinol.

To fully understand Hormone-D, you need to know the following:

o   Mag RBC

o   Storage Hormone-D (25(OH)D)

o   Active Hormone-D (1,25(OH)D2)

o   Ionized Calcium

o   Potassium RBC (excess Calcium CAUSES Renal Potassium Wasting)

Folks,
It's buried in the research, but the "D"ark side of this Hormone is its ability to CRASH Potassium and INCREASE unbound Iron due to its negative affect on Ceruloplasmin (Cp) production in the

Liver...

This LOSS of Cp goes on to affect scores of enzymes and metabolic pathways that are vital to our health and well-being, not the least of which is ATP production (given its role in activating cytochrome C oxidase enzyme in Complex IV of the mitochondria) AND ALL Anti-Oxidant Enzymes... (This is the OTHER side to WHY high Calcitriol >>> Increased Inflammation...)

This was a GREAT thread, and I learned tons... I just hope MORE MAG-pies can wake up to the "D"eception surrounding this supplement...

WHOLEFOOD C: FACTORS TO CONSIDER

Whole food vitamin C brands. The use of whole food vitamin C supports the Liver's production of Ceruloplasmin (Cp), and the Adrenals need for WHOLE C Complex - both providing bio-available Copper...

Among the best brands providing wholefood Vit-C Complex:

o   Innate Response
o   Alive!
o   Grown by Nature
o   Garden of Life
o   MegaFood
o   Standard Process
o   Professional Research Labs

Whole food vitamin C has to be prepared in a low heat process to protect viability. Camu camu, acerola cherry rosehips and sumac are four other whole food, not processed, sources. Please be sure to verify that these frequently "powdered" forms of WF Vit-C have NO ascorbic acid!

http://www.realvitaminc.com/ascorbic-acid.html
http://gotmag.org/ascorbic-acid-causes-Copper-deficiency.../

We need to move beyond the notion of "one mineral <> one enzyme function" That is PURE BIG Pharma "D"eception.

Please note the reach of Cu Deficiency here:

http://www.ncbi.nlm.nih.gov/m/pubmed/2539851/

The blockbuster book by Andre Voisin, "Soil, Grass, Cancer" (1957) made it VERY clear to me, that bioavailable Copper is

KEY to optimal Catalase function. The health of the Anti-Oxidant Enzymes (SOD, CAT, GSH) is a function of the health of Copper, which is BEST determined by the health of Ceruloplasmin (Cp) and the Iron metabolism THAT IT REGULATES...

Please know, Ascorbic Acid is NOT an Anti-oxidant... Look it up on any ORAC table... it is PRO-Oxidant.

That has been PURE "D"eception to call Ascorbic Acid an "anti-oxidant..." ONLY in its **wholefood**, **natural** and **complete** form is Vitamin-C an Anti-oxidant, and it's one of the MOST important in terms of its role in MANAGING Iron in the body...

SYNTHETIC SUPPLEMENTS

It's always important to consider the source of the supplement...

Synthetics work very differently than MTHR NATURE. Beef liver is a perfect balance of Zn<>Cu<>Fe... Yes, it contains ALL 3, and we don't balk at downing that all in one fell swoop... And this is true of pumpkin seeds, and many other natural, food sources of these vital minerals.

All bets are off when it comes to synthetics...

The form of supplements that you're taking are Whole Food concentrates... combining them should not present any issues, as you are eating food...

METABOLIC
FACTORS

ADRENAL FATIGUE

Here's and interesting article about Ceruloplasmin dysfunction and AF "it appears that Cp dysfunction, rather than its absolute plasma levels, may play a major aetiological role in AF, and in turn that Cp dysfunction can be due to **genetic mutation** or oxidative stress (ie after bypass surgery, diabetes, increased levels of H2O2 etc)."

http://onlinelibrary.wiley.com/doi/10.1111/joim.12156/pdf

Ceruloplasmin dysfunction: a key factor in the pathophysiology of atrial fibrillation? With primary emphasis on "genetic mutation."

http://onlinelibrary.wiley.com/doi/10.1111/joim.12156/pdf

OMg!

MAG me with a spoon!...

Our Adrenals are taking a hammering. Let's TOTALLY ignore the fact that we've been "D"rowning in:

o   Ca supplements that hose Maggie and INCREASE "Stress!", increase Stress Hormones, and thereby SLOWS / STOP Cp production...

o   Fe supplements that CAUSE Oxidative Stress to the Cu ions, and thus the structure and functionality of the Cp molecule...

o   Ascorbic Acid, NOT Wholefood Vit-C, that when mixed with XS Iron, creates an Oxidative STORM -- see above ^^^...

o   "D" only supplements that hose Retinol (Vit-A), a KEY precursor to the production of Ceruloplasmin...

o   HFCS (CAUSES a drop in Liver Copper and a RISE in Liver Iron) thus LOWERING the mineral REQUIRED to make Cp, and correspondingly ELEVATING the mineral that OXIDIZES Cp...

o   The hyper-promotion of a LOW-FAT diet that LOWERS the absorption of Copper, the very mineral needed to make Cp...

o   GMO Everything that targets Copper and Magnesium removal -- among others -- from the soil, the plant and the digester of same... (I'll let you connect the dots on that ^^^...)

o   The toxic effect of Fluoride (found in ~75% of all manipulated water) on the function of Cp metabolism... and

o   The ubiquitous presence of Chloride, especially in our water, that alters the conformational structure of Cp...

o   AND THOSE ARE JUST THE "D"ICTUMS THAT HAVE SURFACED, TO DATE...

Yes, let's PRETEND that we're "broken" and have a genetic "D"efect that prevents us from making Cp on our own...

It's ever so much more palatable to our belief system that we're RULED by genes...

Let's NOT own up to the FACT that our Mineral Denialist idiopaths, and their colleagues in the Food System, have been PROMOTING the very "D"ietary "D"ictums that "D"ecrease and

"D"istort optimal Cp production INSIDE our Liver...

How "D"umb do they think we are?!?...

And more importantly, how "D"etached from reality have we been, having been corralled into these "D"ietary "D"istortions over the last 75 years of programming?...

This article, in a word, is offensive and will be taken down in the morning! My only regret is that MORE people won't take the time to read this article and these relevant comments -- they're too busy worrying about their Thyroid #'s, their Iron status and LOW Vit-D...

OMg!... (This is classic "Wizard of Oz" -- pay NO attention to the man behind the curtain!...)

Despite my rant, thank you for posting this provocative article!...

Folks, knowing what I know about the VITAL importance of wholefood Vit-C and healthy Adrenals, you might find this a more cost-effective approach:

http://davesgarden.com/guides/articles/viewith3126/#b

I would advise you STAY AWAY from ANY form of Ascorbic Acid, even Liposomal Vitamin-C, as it does NOT strengthen the production of Ceruloplasmin, NOR the Adrenals...

RDI of Ascorbic Acid = 1,000 mgs...
RDI of Wholefood Vit-C = 60mgs...

You likely will need ~800mgs of WF Vit-C to offset the imbalances in your Cu/Fe metabolism...

The ONLY issue to worry about that I know of, is "increased recovery!"

The Adrenal Glands are involved to the extent you are a "Stress! Cadet"... HIGH "Stress!" and the corresponding elevations of Cortisol ZAP Cp production in the Liver. That is why Maggie is soooo important to have at Optimal levels to ensure our "chill factor!"

Bodies do NOT go into "Fight or Flight!" by accident...

There is a biological REASON for that dynamic:

http://www.ncbi.nlm.nih.gov/pmc/articles/PMC3198864/

The KEY is to identify WHAT is causing the Mg Loss in your body... What I am learning with increasing fervor is that excess, unmanaged Iron, in alleged "anemic" bodies, is a PRIME source of this mg-depleting dynamic...

When was the last time to you assessed the following:

http://requestatest.com/mag-zinc-copper-panel-with-iron-panel-testing

Where there is metabolic dysfunction, there is mineral deficiency and dysregulation...

This is where ALL the symptoms begins...

AGING PROCESS

Here's a VERY different model of aging, but one that HONORS our biology, and NOT the booga-wooga, "you're getting older" mantra...

o Bioavailable Copper is ESSENTIAL for ALL enzymes needed to break down offensive chemicals, i.e. amines, phenols, etc.

o Copper is MADE bioavailable by PROPER amounts of Ceruloplasmin (Cp) which is made principally in the Liver, and the brain...

o MOST "D"aily "D"ietary "D"ictums are "D"esigned to SHUT DOWN the Liver's production of this KEY enzyme...

o Iron is ALSO made bioavailable by PROPER amounts of Cp!

o It's worth noting that Ceruloplasmin is ALSO very sensitive to Oxidative Stress!...

o It's a KNOWN fact in research circles that Cp "ages" due to Oxidative Stress!...

o Two KEY sources of "aging" Ceruloplasmin:

   - lack of sufficient Cp production in the Liver...
   - too much unbound Iron which CREATES Oxidative Stress!...

It is the "AGING" of our Ceruloplasmin in our Liver that is the Culprit -- not the vacuous, I can't do anything about it, so called aging process...

A sure sign that the Liver is "Aging" are the SPOTS we obtain, on our face, arm and hands as we age...

Au contraire to the social meme of aging!... There IS something that we can ALL do about producing proper amounts of Ceruloplasmin and in turn, connect the Iron function throughout our bodies...

CERULOPLASMIN

Folks-- Please understand that I KNOW how confusing this is...

If you DON'T know your Copper/Ceruloplasmin status and are focusing on Iron supplementation -- particularly based on a questionable, solitary Iron protein (Ferritin), it is FAR MORE likely that you are creating the breeding ground for Oxidative Stress!, which is manifested as Allopecia (hair loss...)

ALL is NOT as it seems... Please know that!

Lack of proper Ceruloplasmin (Cp) production in the Liver, is a Cu-dependent process that requires ~20 factors to ensure optimal levels of production...

I can't speak for the SpectraCell testing as it offers NO specific nutrient levels in its reports, but only a given nutrient relative to their unprovided reference ranges...

I regularly work with HTMAs and this blood test (below) to assist clients correct their perceptions and imbalances re their Copper issues:

http://requestatest.com/mag-zinc-Copper-panel-with-Iron-ferritin-test/

(It is worth noting that Bill Walsh, PhD got his start interpreting HTMAs many moons ago...)

The object is NOT to "D"etox Copper, but to STIMULATE the production of Ceruloplasmin (Cp) in your Liver. If you do not know your Cp level, it's an exercise in futility to correct this Copper dynamic. The consequence can be severe...

Do you know your level of Ceruloplasmin (Cp)?... Do you know your levels of Zn, Cu and Fe?...Do you know your Iron levels from a FULL Iron panel, and not a simple ferritin test?

The object is NOT to "chelate" Copper, but enhance the production of Cp in the Liver, thereby increasing the bio-availability of that Copper...

High Copper is missing its anti-oxidant partner, Ceruloplasmin, which is TOTALLY lost on most practitioners and writers addressing the dynamics of this VITAL mineral...

When you solve the Ceruloplasmin (Cp) issue, you address BOTH Copper and Iron dynamics. Keep in mind, Cp requires 8 Copper ions to MAKE IT, 4 of which are Cupric, AND 4 of which are Cuprous...

Cp plays PROFOUND roles in the body besides just shuttling Copper and Iron around. It is a 1st line anti-oxidant that is completely overlooked by, MOST conventional practitioners...

As for the soil issue, Andre Voisin wrote a wonderful book, "Soil, Grass, Cancer" in 1957. It is a mind-numbing account about the LACK OF COPPER in the soil causing a LACK OF COPPER in the grass, causing a LACK OF COPPER in the Cow, causing a LACK OF COPPER in the human, and there by causing a LACK OF COPPER in our cells TO FIGHT CANCER...

Getting access to "proper Copper" is exciting, but we STILL need to make optimal levels of Ceruloplasmin -- for many reasons, not the least of which is to make Copper and Iron USABLE inside the cell...

To take on the fields of Agriculture, Pharmaceuticals and Medicine seems a bit lavish. Know that "Improper" Copper ($Cu2+$) is being used -- and has been used for the last century -- for very specific reasons. Little chance that we will turn that tide.

But what we CAN DO, is gain increased access to "proper Copper," make Mo' Cp, and get off the grid off convention...

And if you're NOT consuming sufficient quantities of Retinol, animal-based Vitamin-A, it will have the SAME effect of lowering the production of Ceruloplasmin in the Liver, thereby lowering your level of Bioavailable Copper, thereby lowering your levels of anti-oxidant enzymes (SOD, and CAT, especially) and thereby INCREASING your hair loss due to the increased Oxidative Stress!...

With all due respect, we would be FAAAR better off seeing a Veterinarian for these types of mineral imbalances:

http://www.tennesseemeatgoats.com/articles2/Copperdeficiency.html

When we have multiple signs and symptoms of LOW bioavailable Copper, we need to take pro-active steps to address thats. Know that Anti-biotics, as a class of drug are designed to BIND UP COPPER!...

That is NOT in anyone's best interest...

Yes, some additional opinions and perspectives seem warranted.

Weak Adrenals = LOW production of Ceruloplasmin in Liver = HIGH amount of unbound Copper...

HIGH UNbound Copper = LOW bound ("proper") Copper = LOW Cytochrome C Oxidase (Mitochondria Complex IV) = LOW ATP = LOW Energy!

THAT'S the metabolic mechanism...

Signs/symptoms of LOW Bioavailable Copper (Copper LACKING Ceruloplasmin...)

o   UTI's -- insufficient CuZnSOD to kill the pathogenic bacteria...

o   Migraines -- inability to activate DAO, MAO and/or HNMT enzymes that are designed to break down Histamines that CAUSE Migraines...

o   Alzheimer's -- insufficient CuZnSOD to NEUTRALIZE the Oxidative Stress CAUSED by Aluminum and Iron that build up when Copper is NOT bioavailable...

Please know that the world is overflowing with folks who are dealing with excess, bioUN-available Copper due to a systemic INABILITY to produce Ceruloplasmin as they actually listened to their Mineral Denialists and Dieticians about what supplements to take...

Just in case you have been living under a rock or a newbie - MAGpie:

Here are the steps to Increase Ceruloplasmin (Cp):

o   STOP Hormone-D ONLY Supplements (KILLS Liver Retinol needed for Cp)

o   STOP Calcium Supplements! (Ca BLOCKS Mg and Iron absorption...)
o   STOP Iron Supplements! (Fe SHUTS DOWN Cu metabolism...)

o   STOP Ascorbic Acid (It disrupts the Copper<>Cp bond)

- o STOP HFCS and Synthetic Sugars (HFCS Lowers Liver Copper)

- o STOP LOW Fat Diet (Fat is needed for proper Copper absorption)

- o STOP Using Industrialized, "Heart Healthy" Oils!

- o STOP Using products with Fluoride (toothpaste, bottled Water, etc.)

- o STOP Taking "Mulit's" and "Pre-natals" (They have 1st four items ^^^^)

- o START CLO (1 tsp Rosita's or 1 TBSP Nordic Naturals) for Retinol (Vit-A)

- o START Mg supps to lower ACTH and Cortisol (Dose: 5mgs/lb body weight)

- o START Wholefood Vit-C (500-800 mgs/day) - source of Copper

- o START B8 (Biotin) -- Key for Cu/Fe regulation in Liver

- o START B2 (Riboflavin) -- Key for Cu/Fe regulation in Liver

- o START Boron -- 1-3 mgs/day (aids in Synthesis of Cp)

- o START Taurine to support Copper metabolism in the Liver

- o START Ancestral Diet (HIGH Fat and Protein/LOW Carb)

o   START Iodine (PREQUISITE: Mg and Se RBC need to be optimal)

Please note, the first 9 Steps are what doctors and nutritionists have been GUIDING us TO DO for the last 75 years...

Hmmmmmmmmm....

Yes, these co-factors noted ^^^^ are very important, although I'm no longer "bullish" on "B"ottled B's...

I much prefer folks get them from food:

o   Bee Pollen (I love the fact that MTHR NATURE has Bee's providing us with "B's!")

o   Stabilized Rice Bran

o   Nutritional Yeast -- yes, I'm aware of the "supplementation of "Folic Acid"-- I've got a call with the chief scientist at Bragg's to discuss this on Monday...

o   "Bee"f Liver -- grass-fed and grass-finished, of course...

Finally, while you may have a hard time finding this on a "Google search," I'm increasingly of the opinion that Copper is KEY to the activation of B-vitamins... (It plays that role in ALL Biogenic amines)

This activation process is SUPPOSED to occur in our gut. And how did I come to this weird conclusion?...

ALL forms of natural B's are joined with Copper... I don't think that's an accident.

And, just to stir the pot.... what about those with blocked pathways that can't convert even wholefood B's?

http://www.healthaliciousness.com/articles/foods-high-in-riboflavin-vitamin-B2.php

http://www.whfoods.com/genpage.php?tname=nutrientanddbid=42

Blocked pathways are almost ALWAYS from a lack of bioavailable Copper that prevents proper Methylation of the B's...

It is a process... I just think an entire couple of generations have been "trained" to "B"elieve that those vittles form from the "B"ottle are exactly the "same" as those from REAL FOOD. Nothing could be FARTHER from the truth...

Additional Factors to consider re Ceruloplasmin:

o   Chlorinated water is very hard on Cp production...

o   High dose Zinc supplements BLOCK Copper absorption...

Please note that the first 9 "STOPS!" are what our doctors and nutritionists have been telling us TO DO for the last 75 years...

Lack of sufficient Cp CAUSES:

o   LOW Iron absorption (serum Iron) >> 57 -- it should be ~100

o   HIGH Transferrin >> 410 -- It should be ~285

o   LOW Iron saturation (Fe/TIBC) >> 14% -- It should be ~33%

o   LOWish Hemoglobin... it's Copper dependent, especially the need for Ferrochelatase to place Iron in the Hemoglobin molecule.

o   HIGH UNbound Copper that is affecting the production of KEY Anti-Oxidant Enzymes (SOD, CAT, GSH)

Regrettably, there are 20 factors -- and counting -- that must be addressed to optimize Cp production. And while folks who take wholefood Vit-C, CLO, Maggie, natural B's may not get immediate Cp improvement, it might ALSO have to do with the presence of:

o   Fluoride
o   Chloride
o   Citrate molecule (ubiquitous presence in processed food...)
o   Iron supplements
o   Zinc supplements -- it KILLS Cp production, by BLOCKING Copper absorption!...
o   Multi-vitamins and Pre-Natals that violate ALL the STOPS!
o   and a whole host of other factors...

Regrettably, Cp is OUTRAGEOUSLY important, and falls on DEAF ears in the worlds of both conventional medicine and natural healing.

As you discover more and more about this protein/enzyme, there are some and KNOWN impacts:

o   Copper metabolism,
o   Iron metabolism,
o   Biogenic Amine (neurotransmitters and vitamins) metabolism,
o   Energy metabolism,
o   Anti-Oxidant Enzyme metabolism,
o   Activation of Oxidase enzymes
o   To name JUST a few key pathways... your jaw will drop

as you wonder HOW this CRITICAL ENZYME was suppressed in clinical training...

We're quickly going to get into a chicken<>egg dynamic...

Yes, the transcription error is real, but it AIN'T in concrete. And that's a fact. Yes, there clearly is a very real issue here, but what I'm learning is that the IRON side of the house needs to be in order, as well... There are multiple facets to Iron Metabolism -- ALL REQUIRE Ceruloplasmin...

Ceruloplasmin (Cp) is the link between these two oxidizing minerals, as you well know... It is likely one of the MOST important, and LEAST understood, proteins on the Planet... by design, mind you...

Regrettably, faaaaaar too many folks have gotten HOSED by taking excess Hormone-D supplements which has a "D"ecidedly chilling affect on the production of Cp. And THAT'S a fact...

Faaaaar too many folks have been "D"rowning their bodies with Ascorbic Acid -- for generations!...

Faaaaar too many folks have been believing the BS re the need for Iron supplements, and thinking that they've got "Iron poor blood" -- NOT knowing that Iron supplements KILL Copper metabolism and thus the production of Cp...

Faaaaar too many folks have wickedly LOW Maggie status that dramatically affects the Liver's ability to make this key enzyme, as excess Cortisol, borne from Mg deficiency, STOPS Cp production...

And I could go on...

Yes, the EPIGENETIC factors are, in fact, what CAUSED this gene transcription error. It is a body ADAPTING TO STRESS -- the stress of Copper dysregulation, borne of a toxic food system,

171

and mis-directed medical system, BOTH OF WHOM have gone out of their way to bring our Livers to their knees!...

There is NOT ONE neurogenerative condition that is NOT borne of the dysregulation of BOTH Iron and Copper metabolism. And the protein/enzyme that gets FAAAAAAR too little attention is Ceruloplasmin. Call me crazy, but I refuse to believe that the Liver will NOT respond when properly AND completely stimulated by the correct levels of nutrients...

Again, genes transcription errors are JUST LIKE circuit breakers in your home... they DO flip back!...But the "Stressors!" Need to be connected.

When Ceruloplasmin is being UNDER-produced in the Liver, it creates two simultaneous and inter-acting events:

o   Low bioavailable Copper... => Lack of Anti-Oxidant Enzymes (SOD, CAT, GSH)

o   High mismanaged Iron... => Abundance of Oxidative "Stress!" (ROS=Reactive Oxygen Species)

Hmmmmmm...

I wonder if THAT'S covered in conventional clinical training?...

Help me understand how adding Zinc will help in the production of Cp... In studies that I've read, the Ferroxidase activity of Cp goes down to "0" five days following the intake of Zinc...

My position is MOST sincere...

I simply do NOT understand the "Take Zinc to improve your Cp" mantra. Clearly, I'm missing something VERY basic, or they do NOT understand Cp pharology.

And what my relentless reading and reflection is revealing is that

NOT ALL Cp is the same... There is "Active" and "Inactive" Cp. And the "Active" has Ferroxidase activity and the "Inactive" does NOT. And THAT'S a BIG DEAL...

I'll look forward to your thoughts and suggestions on what to consider or what else to read...

All this foment over "Free" Copper is unnecessary...

I take the Cp level and multiply by three to identify the level of USABLE Copper.

The closer that number of USABLE copper is to 100, the better.

The caveat is that Cp elevates with:

o   Pregnancy
o   Birth Control Pill use
o   Inflammation and
o   Infection

Cp measured in a blood test tells us how much protein is STRUCTURALLY = to Cp. The standard blood test tells us NOTHING about the ENZYMATIC POTENCY of this critical protein.

They make this distinction ALL THE TIME in research studies, and aparently, do NOT allow its measurement commercially.

WHY, you ask?!?

If you knew how LOW the enzyme function of your Cp was, then you'd KNOW how at risk you were for the TOTAL mismanagement of your Iron metabolism, and its corresponding impact on increasing your Oxidative "Stress!"

Can't have THAT, now can we?!?...

Please, move your focus on creating bioavailable Cp and ease off your "booga-wooga Copper" focus... Copper is NOT the bad guy. You have 23X MORE IRON than Copper in your body and THAT mineral (Fe) is profoundly involved in creating Oxidative Stress!

You are LOW in bioavailable Copper and HIGH in unmanaged Iron... And the CAUSE is LOW Cp production in your Liver...

Properly raised animal Liver for human consumption, is among the MOST nutrient dense foods on the Planet. You have been programmed to think it ONLY has Iron, when it has a proper balance of Copper and Zinc, Cp and a 6oz serving has 20,000 IUs of Retinol. (That would be the amount needed <u>EVERY TIME</u> you take two drops of synthetic, soy-based Hormone-D...)

As for Beta-carotene, it is just MORE "D"ietary "D"eception. It takes 12 Beta-carotene + Zn + ENERGY to equal 1 molecule of Retinol. Our Livers, by the way, RUN on Retinol..

And when you "D"rown yourself in "D"-only supplements, the Retinol RUNS AWAY, which STOPS the production of Ceruloplasmin (Cp)...

Yes, THAT'S why they are pushing sooooo hard to "D"eceive you...

Cp is It's one of the MOST important proteins/enzymes you've NEVER heard of...

After all, no $$$$ in a cure!...

Earl Frieden, PhD, at the University of Florida, Gainesville, was likely among the most lucid Copper researchers about the importance of Ceruloplasmin in the human body:

http://www.ncbi.nlm.nih.gov/pmc/articles/PMC2195460/

http://www.ncbi.nlm.nih.gov/pubmed/775938

http://www.sciencedirect.com/science/article/pii/S096800047680
1314

Please note the dates of his research precede the distortion of reality ushered into medical research during the Reagan Administration...

Not sure what further needs to be said. Cp brings good things to LIFE!...

CHOLESTEROL

At the risk of offending those precious few on MAG who actually think that their allopathic sherpas have their "best" interests "at least", the medical machine is doing to Ceruloplasmin what it did to Cholesterol, for the past 60 years -- "D"emonize it!...

The scale of the offense and scientific sleight of hand is mind-numbing...

There are precious few lipids that are MORE important than Cholesterol...

In like fashion, there are precious few Proteins/Enzymes that are MORE important than Ceruloplasmin (Cp)...

Here's a PARTIAL List of what Cp does:

o   Primary Copper transport protein

o   Lipid Anti-Oxidant Activity (see my comments re Lipid
        Peroxidation below...)

o   Primary agent for Iron Homeostasis via it's CRITICAL role
        of Oxidizing Ferrous (2+)   >> Ferric (3+) Iron -- THAT IS
        A MAJOR EVENTinside the body, by the way...)

o   Primary agent for the Oxidation of "Biogenic Amines" like
        Dopamine, Noradrenaline, Adrenaline, Seratonin,
        Thyroxine (Please let that Cp role sink in for a moment...
        these "amines" do NOT work until *KISSED*   by Cp...
        Hmmmmmm... Know anyone in your circle of
        family/friends with any issues re ANY of these
        "amines?!?"...)

o   Energy metabolism... Cytochrome c Oxidase in

Complex IV of the ETC inside the Mitochondria, too, must get kissed by Cp...

o   Anti-Oxidant Enzyme Metabolism... SOD will NOT work without Cp...

o   Regulates Hypoxia Inducible Factor-1 (HIF-1) -- another BIG deal in Oxygen and Iron REGULATION...

o   Glutathione-Peroxidase activity is Cp dependent... (Said another way, Glutathione does NOT work without Cp...)

o   Bactericidal Activity...

o   Coagulation of blood as the Amino Acid profile of Cp mirrors that of Factors V and VIII in the blood...

o   Primary defense against Oxidant Stress! in the blood and tissue...

And that's what I've figured out Part-time between the ongoing pace of HTMA consults... (Think what I could amass were I JUST devoted to this quixotic Cp quest FULL-TIME!... ;-))

And instead of medical researchers telling us that Cholesterol is the GATEWAY to Steroid Hormone production via its natural CONVERSION into Pregnenalone, as a world community, we were HELD HOSTAGE for 60+ years of TOTAL scientific fiction while BIG Pharma amassed BILLION$ upon BILLION$ stuffing us with $tatin$ to "treat" this alledged un-toward, evil molecule in our body...

(And what THEY forgot to tell us is that, in fact, the LACK of BIOAVAILABLE Copper (due to missing Cp!!!!) is what CAUSES the Lipid Peroxidation that becomes the very Plaque of our fears... Know that unbound Iron is MOST effective at stimulating Lipid Peroxidation, aka "Plaque")

And NOW, what we are being assaulted with is, Ceruloplasmin is an "Acute Phase Reactive Protein" and is "booga-wooga!" OMg! MAG me with a spoon!!!

"Fool me once, shame on THEM... Fool me twice, shame on US... "

And what is ESSENTIAL for Cp production are TWO primary components:

o   Copper ions; and

o   Retinoic Acid (derived from Retinol, when the Liver is NOT being "D"rowned in Calcitriol, also known as Vit- D... Hmmmmmmmm...)

And so we're bring "TRAINED" -- like Circus Bears -- to treat Copper as the enemy and "D"rown it with Zinc. Zinc has an immediate effect on BLOCKING Copper absorption, thus decreasing Cp production.

Furthermore, what is fascinating is that Metallothionein, another KEY Metalloenzyme, is made with EIGHT (8) Zinc ions and holds onto Copper 1,000 MORE strongly than Ceruloplasmin. WOW!

So, please forgive the blah, blah, blah ^^^^... This is WAAAAAY more complicated than we realize and WAAAAAY more convoluted than the pedestrian Internet articles on Copper would have us believe.

CORTISOL

The status of Potassium is considered a surrogate measurement for Cortisol on the HTMA... I'm not aware of a specific marker; although I seem to recall some research last year alluding to that as a test.

My focus would be more directed at the role of Copper deficiency in affecting Phospholipid status. Fig 2 of the 2nd article below is worth the price of admission:

http://pubag.nal.usda.gov/pubag/downloadPDF.xhtml?id=47546a ndcontent=PDF 2)

http://ajcn.nutrition.org/content/48/3/637.full.pdf

Mg is KEY to recycling Cortisol BACK to its storage form, CORTISONE... as well as for ensuring proper Circadian Rhythm that dictates the Cortisol levels throughout the day...

http://www.ncbi.nlm.nih.gov/pmc/articles/PMC3327520/pdf/74010 16.pdf

You might take a copy of that article to your doctor... they might actually learn how the body REALLY works!...

Mg turns OFF the Sympathetic "Stress!" Response. Mg, also plays a key role in the production of Cortisol via its activation of the enzyme family responsible for creating ALL hormones. Mg also activates the key enzyme that recycles Cortisol (active state) back to Cortisone (storage state). Technically, it's more accurate to say that Mg "regulates" Cortisol...

The fact that you're concerned with low Cortisol means your

Potassium level is low, likely due to excess, unbound Copper and/or Iron. Please know that you cannot restore Potassium until Mg levels are optimal, and Retinol plays an important role to "prime" the Potassium pump.

I would strongly advise a Mag RBC and an HTMA to assess your mineral status overall...

http://www.gotmag.org/work-with-us/

EMOTIONAL STATE

Emotional state AND Thyroid Function are RULED by Mineral status, levels and ratios...

Sorry, it's time we END the insanity that the Thyroid "rules" the body!...

Please know, at the base of ALL that you speak of are Mineral imbalances and dysregulation, both of which affect enzyme functions that then go on to make Hormones...

It is NOT Hormone imbalance, the stree-induced mineral imbalance precedes it EVERY TIME!!!...

This is NOT an insignificant point of clarification. What we are teaching here at MAG is that "Stressors!" affect our mineral status, notably Maggie and Copper, in particular. The cascade of imbalances from JUST those two minerals inside the body and inside the cells is mind-numbing...

This is very well addressed in this classic article:

http://www.ncbi.nlm.nih.gov/pmc/articles/PMC3198864/

That article should be taught and LEARNED in the 1st week of Medical School... It's THAT Basic and THAT Foundational to our well being and health...

Hormones, Tissue tears and Tiredness ALL relate to Copper dysregulation... the Achilles Heel of HTMA analysis is the interpretation of Copper status, regrettably... That is why I do targeted blood testing to get to the TRUTH of your Copper and Iron metabolisms:

o   Mag RBC
o   Plasma Zinc
o   Serum Copper...
o   Serum Ceruloplasmin...
o   Serum Iron...
o   Serum Transferrin...
o   Serum TIBC (% sat)
o   Serum Ferritin...

Yes, it requires a Full Monty view of these metals to UNDERSTAND the dynamics of Copper and Iron, particularly given their siamese Twin relationship to Ceruloplasmin...

EXERCISE

Movement is the key... Hard cardio is best pursued by those seeking to deplete their "Mineral Buckets!"...

Please know, I've completed 3 Marathons, 1/2 dozen Half-Marathons and 1 Olympic-Distance Triathlon...

It is only by the Grace of God, that when my upper thighs (Quads and Hamstrings) LOCKED UP in the last stage of that last event, that I didn't keel over grabbing my chest...

It's in part due to THAT close call that I reached new levels of passion about the importance of these minerals (and Maggie, of course...) and became a MAG-piper!...

The key for MAG-pies is that on those days when you awake to: "I'm feeling so much better," you exercise caution and try NOT to climb Mt. Everest (at least not without a team of Sherpas...)

All too many MAG-pies have made that understandable mistake... Easy does it...

Remember, Maggie is the mineral of motion... not the mineral of mountain climbing...

As much as we seek the "Killer App!" -- it doesn't exist... based on our experience, there are some obvious "To Do's," and some "NOT To Do's," but at the end of the day, each of us must experiment and assess what form(s) of Maggie and other minerals work BEST in our bodies...

And in a perfect world, that effort would be based on mineral testing to know the expected impact of our efforts...

FOOD

Eat for Your Blood Type is a Guide, it is NOT the Gospel...
Equally as important are:

o   Eating a seasonal diet of REAL food...
o   Eating locally and organically...
o   Eating the foods that your Ancestors ate -- your DNA is
       programmed to THOSE nutrients due to millennia of
       generations of programming...

Cows are DESIGNED to eat and process grass -- NOT GMO
Corn and GMO Soy -- and are designed to turn it into products
that are good for us. However, having them eat even "Organic"
Corn and Soy is NOT "OK!" It is NOT natural, despite it being
"Organic!"

As a society that has LOST touch with the land, we have
TOTALLY lost our connection with how animals are to be fed,
ALLOWED to graze in the SUNSHINE!, and let their perfectly
designed metabolisms create a saturated fat, that has sustained
people for millennia of millennia...

So, if the Cows are eating "Organic" grass -- Heaven forbid! --
then we're cool...

Please know, the word "Organic" is one of the MOST abused
and "D"istorted words in the field of Food MARKETING... We
respond like Pavlovian "D"ogs when we see it, and FAIL to
question -- WHAT IS ACTUALLY "ORGANIC" IN WHAT I AM
ABOUT TO EAT?!?...

May you live in "interesting" times...
(-- Famous Chinese Curse!)

In case you didn't know it, we are being POISONED by the food, pharmaceutical and medical systems...

The human metabolism is under assault and apparently they don't teach that in the advanced academic programs in the U.K....

All is NOT as it seems...

And I commend you for choosing to be an organic farmer. More folks need to adopt that level of commitment.

Regrettably, most folks lack the land, and even more lack the options in the food markets to gain access to unadulterated foods...

Please track down and read this important book by Andre Voisin, a dairy farmer from the U.K: "Soil, Grass, Cancer" published in 1957.

It will open your eyes to the REAL story of agriculture, and HOW NPK was DESIGNED to change the plants access to vital minerals so that humans would NOT have access to same...

Again, ALL is NOT as it seems...

Word to the wise...

Turn "Smoothies" >>> "Chewsies" by adding seeds, nuts, etc. to ensure the use of our TEETH, the chewing function that activates the Parotid Glands, which then in turn releases Amylase enzyme designed to break down the abundance of carbs in these breakfast drinks...

Please note: Digestion STARTS with chewing, NOT swallowing...

Good point, and this also applies for those with digestive issues, as well...

My veiled point ^^^, given that I'm TOTALLY into Ancestral Nutrition, is that, to my knowledge, Weston A. Price, DDS and his wife Isabelle, found NO blenders in their decade-long search for the perfect diet to create perfect teeth...

The fact that they are popular is NOT a guarantee that they are not necessarily good for our health...

Ancestral grains have nutrients that have sustained us for 10,000 years...

Weaponized grains due to pre-harvest spraying with (Glyphosate) arrived just 30 years ago...

https://nourishingourchildren.wordpress.com/2015/05/12/the-nourishing-traditions-cookbook-for-children/

They deserve, but will never get, a Pulitzer for this!... it's a cornerstone in ALL sane kitchens around the Globe.

What is sobering however is that there are 7+Billions residents on this Blue Marble hurling through space... To date, a little over 400,000 have purchased this wonderful book...
It makes an AMAZING Birthday or holiday gift!...
You can buy a used copy for <$15.00
http://www.amazon.com/gp/offer-listing/0967089735/ref=sr_1_1_twi_1_pap_olp?s=books&ie=UTF8&qid=1431812444&sr=1-1&keywords=nourishing%20traditions%20sally%20fallon

GENES

I would suggest that most, if not all, so-called "gene mutations" are from excess, unmanaged Iron created during 3-4 generations of hyper Iron-fortified foods eaten by organisms that are BOTH Mg deficient AND lack Bioavailable Copper/Ceruloplasmin...

Flood the body with Toxic levels of Iron, and "steal away" their Cu and Mg (to regulate and manage it) and the actions of enzymes change dramatically -- due to Iron-induced Oxidative Stress! Even those enzymes designed to REGULATE and REPAIR nucleotide pairs on genes are affected...

Trust me, this AIN'T Rocket Science...

And lest we forget, one of the GREATEST "Stressors!" that gets overlooked is:

Iron "Stress!"

http://ghr.nlm.nih.gov/gene/SLC40A1

But only those with a recognition of Copper/Cp can understand this concept, n'est ce pas?!?...

Assess your Copper and Ceruloplasmin (Cp) status and see what you are doing to BLOCK the Liver's production of Cp, and what you can do to STIMULATE same with proper diet and supplements...

Yes, I'm well aware of the "belief system" that HH (human hemochromatosis) is "caused" by a mutation of the HFE gene... Maybe so, maybe not.

The Liver's been on this Planet a LOOOOOONG time. Give it the nutrients to work its MAG-ic and STOP abusing it with stuff like synthetic, soy-based hyper-vitaminosis-D, as well as Iron-fortified flour and stand back!

Know that Hepcidin is REGULATED by Ceruloplasmin, despite only a select few Iron researchers who well note this metabolic reality...

http://www.sciencedirect.com/science/article/pii/S092544390700 2396

I totally agree with your sentiments re gov'l "meddling," especially their TOTAL violation of "informed consent," and our implicit "trust" that govt's exist to **protect**, NOT **poison** their subjects...

Silly us for thinking like sovereigns with inalienable rights... ;-)

I'll stick to MTHR NATURE to promote Cp production. I'm not a big fan of FTHR TEST TUBE to force production...

Besides, many of the folks I work with are Estrogen dominant, AND Cp anemic... That seems to fly in the face of this study...

CAVEAT READOR!

Please know that "transcription errors," brought to you by epigenetic "Stress!" means that selected enzymes are NOT working for lack of optimal, bioavailable minerals that ACTIVATE these very enzymes...

Be VERY careful how you interpret and respond to the blah, blah, blah of the MTHFR community about these issues...

There is WAAAAAAAY more to the story than what is typically found on most websites that address these booga-wooga mutations, scientifically known as transcription errors...

Yes, these errors need to be understood, but NOT feared. You are NOT broken. And MANY with these issues are fine as they do NOT always express...

It ALL depends on your "Stress!" level and capacity to metabolize "Stress!" -- which is entirely a function of our body's mineral status.

(And I've counted to 100 TWICE so that I don't EXPLODE responding to this added nuance of "D"ietary "D"eception... And it's NOT that you've raised this important question about Hormone-D, it's that ANOTHER nuance of "D"eception needs to be cut down to size... and it AIN'T going to be easy or short...)

Since WWII, MOST people have been ingesting OUTRAGEOUS amounts of Iron, due to "Iron Fortification" programs Worldwide, which are the result of an ENTIRELY constructed belief system that we are ALL "Iron deficient..." *wink!* *wink!*

After all, Iron is the "greatest nutritional deficiency" on the Planet, or so we have been led to believe. Our belief here at MAG in THAT delusion is the underpinning of the entire Allopathetic "D"isease Paradigm...

(Please ignore the FACT that Iron is the 3rd most abundant element on Earth, factoring out Oxygen as #1... We, as a species, MUST believe that we are "Iron deficient..." and that we have LOST the innate capacity to properly handle Iron that MILLIONS of our Ancestors had before us...)

Adding "Iron-y" Insult to "Iron-ic" Injury, manufacturers of food and supplement products have played a carnival shell game about how much Iron we are ACTUALLY getting in our food... Truth be known, the average adult needs by the way 6-8mgs of Iron daily, and when ALL the dust settles with our ridiculous "D"iets, we can get as much as 60-80mgs of Iron EACH AND EVERY DAY depending upon how "processed," "GMO'd" or "HFCS'd" our food happens to be...

To learn MORE about this, please read:
http://freetheanimal.com/2015/06/enrichment-theory-everything.html

Let me be VERY clear -- Iron is vital to our livelihood, but in excess, especially when it becomes 10X our need being ingested DAILY, it is a POISON to our bodies. That Iron excess is THE metabolic engine for CREATING Oxidative Stress!...

It does this flawlessly and tirelessly in our bodies, especially when there is a LACK of Anti-Oxidant Minerals, Vitamins, and Enzymes to neutralize its diabolic effect inside the cell... And know that those enzymes are dependent upon BIOAVAILABLE COPPER for construction and activation...

Now, keep in mind, we are ALL being trained -- LIKE CIRCUS BEARS -- to believe that we have a range of serious nutritional problems that our parents, grandparents and greats NEVER had:

o   Excess Cholesterol, especially LDL -- Note that they FORGOT to tell us that Mg and bioavailable Copper ENSURE optimal production of Cholesterol and ALSO ensure that LCAT enzyme FLIPS LDL >> HDL. Hmmmm... Those are NOT insignificant facts to leave out, but for 60 years we've been held hostage to this silly idea that we have a "Cholesterol disease..." NO, it's just MISSING MINERALS...

o   Vitamin-D Deficiency -- I believe I've made my points on this "D"emonic issue AD NAUSEUM, but what they FORGOT to tell us is that LOW Storage-D means that there's an EXCESS of ACTIVE-D, and this a SHORTAGE OF MAGGIE (they exist on a seesaw together...

Hmmmmm... Another case of MISSING MINERALS...

And that brings us to the so-called "Iron deficiency" "D"ilemma...

191

For over 100 years (1860-1970), Iron Anemia was ALWAYS measured via an assesment of Hemoglobin (potency of Red Blood Cells) and Hematocrit (% of Red Blood Cells), which makes PERFECT sense as 2/3 of our Iron in the body is found in biactive RBCs so that it can provide Oxygen for Oxidative Phosphorylation to make ATP inside our Mitochondria...

But please note the following:

o   you cannot make Heme without bioavailable Copper...

o   You cannot make Hemoglobin without bioavailable Copper...

o   You cannot insert Iron into Hemoglobin without Copper activating Ferrochelatase enzyme...

o   You cannot absorb Iron in your gut without Hephaestin, a Multi-Copper Oxidase Protein...

o   You cannot transport Iron in your blood via Transferrin UNTIL it's *kissed* by a VITAL Copper-dependent protein, Ceruloplasmin...

o   And you cannot make Ferritin store and/or release the excess Iron, unless there are optimal levels of Ceruloplasmin...

Hmmmmmm... Seems like Iron metabolism is COMPLETELY Copper-dependent... (And, in fact, it is...)

Well, one of the GREAT Copper/Iron researchers was Earl Frieden, PhD. He made numerous sterling contributions to the field of Iron metabolism, but a KEY observation appeared in a Nutritional Reviews article in 1970 in which he stated the following:

"Iron accumulates in response to a LACK of active Ceruloplasmin in the circulation."

That is a PROFOUND observation... as Ceruloplasmin is, in my humble opinion, one of the MOST IMPORTANT and LEAST UNDERSTOOD enzymes on this Planet -- (BY METICULOUS "D"ESIGN, mind you)... It is NO accident that we're clueless about this protein/enzyme and that doctors the world over NEVER EVER measure its status, especially when assessing Iron metabolism status...

As Patrick Sullivan Jr. likes to say about Maggie: "It does TOO MUCH!..." Well, the EXACT SAME can be said of Ceruloplasmin. FB lacks sufficient wall space for me to fully delineate ALL that Cp does in our bodies. It is a SIN that we don't know this, but then that's why we're ALL here, right?...

Now, let's turn our focus to the Iron darling, Ferritin. It was discovered in 1937, but it was not until the 1970's that they were able to develop an assay for measuring it accurately in the body. And the concept of "Iron Anemia," as well as measuring "Anemia," was NEVER the same... Out goes the metabolically active measures of Hemoglobin/Hematocrit, and in comes the metabolically INERT measure of storage Iron...(It's akin to assessing what car to buy SOLELY on the size of the trunk, and NOT its pick-up or fuel efficiency!)

Ferritin is a STORAGE protein for Iron that is NOT usable... Each Ferritin molecule can hold up to 1,000 Fe^{+++} atoms. It is there for EXCESS, UNUSABLE IRON, and in a similar fashion to Cholesterol, and Vitamin-D, millions of folks are being TRAINED to believe that it is the sine qua non for assessing "Iron status" in the human body.

TILT NOTHING COULD BE FARTHER FROM THE TRUTH...

What the great Mineral Denialist researchers at Harvard are

193

overlooking is that Hepcidin is dependent on Ceruloplasmin status:

http://www.sciencedirect.com/science/article/pii/S092544391000
1481

Please know, the object of our nutrition of focus on MAG is:

o   NOT to lower Cholesterol to ridiculously LOW levels...

o   NOT to elevate our Storage Hormone-D to ridiculously
      HIGH levels...

o   NOT to elevate our Ferritin to ridiculously HIGH levels --
      completely IGNORING the warnings of enlightened
      Cardiologists the world over that Ferritin >50 is a
      harbinger of Heart Events...

I do apologize for the extended blah, blah, blah... But ONCE
AGAIN, I'm NOT buying the conventional BS re this issue as the
OVERWHELMING MAJORITY of Iron researchers wouldn't know
a Ceruloplasmin molecule if it bit them in the arse... and I have a
SERIOUS problem with their CLINICAL IGNORANCE, as well as
their "D"istorted METABOLIC BELIEF SYSTEM.

In a word, it is FLAWED and it has, and continues to, INJURE
millions and millions of folks on this Planet daily because of a
failure to understand HOW to assess Iron metabolism status and
AVOID EXCESS OXIDATIVE STRESS by limiting the intake of
Iron -- in our diets and our supplement routines -- all for NOT
knowing the regulatory role of Ceruloplasmin in Iron
metabolism....

I have a problem with that "blinded-by-Ferritin" approach, and I'm
dedicating my Mineral Detective efforts to STOP THAT
INSANITY, wherever I can...

Thanks for letting me rant and get some stuff off my chest...

Hope that this comment makes some sense...

Again, please focus on Ceruloplasmin Production... Period!

Ferritin, alone, is hardly the measure of your Iron status...

THE measure of Cp is the Oxidase Activity of Ceruloplasmin. However, it appears NOT to be available publicly.

I'll let you connect the dots why...

And, how do we fix our mitochondrial function?

Complex IV (Cytochrome c Oxidase) doesn't work without bioavailable Copper and Ceruloplasmin (Cp). Iron is structural in that enzyme. If Cu/Cp's missing, the Mitochondria is elegantly designed to make ROS in Complex III...

Hmmmmmm...

Please know, Niacin is a Biogenic amine. They are activated when *kissed* by Cp... This is true of ALL Vital amines and Neurotransmitters. It is conveniently BURIED in the research...

Bottled "B's," and MOST of our clients, do NOT have Cp!...

Now granted, I've only studied carefully 10 of the 200 Methyltransferase enzymes... ALL 10 are dependent on bioavailable Copper.

Please know, that Zinc blocks Copper absorption, as you likely know, but Metallothionein that is triggered by Zinc intake holds onto Copper 1,000X stronger than Zinc...

Hmmmmm...

Methylation requires proper functioning Methytransferase (MT) enzymes...

Of the 10 Methyltransferase (MT) enzymes I've studied carefully (BHMT, COMT, etc.), all 10 of them REQUIRE Copper to properly activate these enzymes... There are 150-200 MT enzymes in the body...

In addition, please know that B-Vitamins are also known as "biogenic amines..." That means that they will NOT work until they are "oxidized" by Ceruloplasmin (Cp), a vital enzyme that requires 8 Copper atoms to work PROPERLY... (Please ignore the current literature that says Cp only needs 6 atoms...)

And what is key to the optimal stereochemical structure of Cp?...

Magnesium!....and it performs a similar role with ATP making that KEY energy chemical usable, as Mg-ATP....

HISTAMINES

When we sprain our ankles, it's always a good idea to stay off that joint and use a crutch to allow time (and MINERALS...) to repair the tissues involved... Interestingly enough, Maggie and Copper are profoundly important in repairing sprains in our ankles -- and our guts, as well soon see ...

Please follow the bouncing balls...

o	The state of Mg deficiency CAUSES an increase in Mast Cells...

https://www.jstage.jst.go.jp/article/jnsv/59/6/59_560/_pdf

(You would be the RATS in the greater global Lab experiment...)

o	Mast Cells are where Histamines are manufactured...

o	Histamines are incredibly important chemicals designed to protect us from our environment, AND they also serve as Neurotransmitters as noted in this wonderful article:

http://ajcn.nutrition.org/content/85/5/1185.full.pdf+html

The REACH of Histamines and Histamine intolerance is WELL expressed in Fig 1 of this wonderful article...

o	What Maintz and Novak seem to OVERLOOK is that two key enzymes are ESSENTIAL to degrade (breakdown) Histamines: DAO and HNMT -- BOTH of which require

Mg, bioavailable Copper and B6. That is NOT an insignificant FACT...

o   MANY, MANY, MANY people on MAG, and on this Planet, do NOT have those three nutrients in sufficient quantities and in proper ratios...

o   In fact, what is increasingly apparent is that MANY have HIGH levels of unbound Copper, which means that it is NOT bioavailable, and thus NOT usable to make DAO, nor to degrade it or its partner enzyme...

o   Furthermore, unbound Copper has a decidedly wicked impact on B-vitamins and Maggie -- it KILLS them! And this is the likely mechanism that prevents an optimal response to either foods that HAVE High Histamines or those that STIMULATE a Histamine response...

o   Histamine Intolerance is a CLASSIC sign of Mg deficiency and Copper dysregulation, in my humble opinion...

So, what to do?...

1)   Get smarter about how your body REALLY works by ignoring 99% of the articles on the web that are written by BIG Pharma, with only ONE objective -- keep you in their clutches...

2)   Get smarter about your overall mineral profile (HTMA) and targeted mineral dynamics of your key metals (Blood test) to learn about the level of production of Ceruloplasmin (Cp) that makes Copper, Iron and

Manganese work inside the body and their interplay endless with Zinc...

3) Get smarter about the 20+ steps needed to improve Ceruloplasmin production in the Liver...

4) Take time off the foods that seem to trigger this "allergic" reaction and work to re-balance your minerals and improve the bioavailability of the key mineral players...

5) Re-assess your mineral status to determine shifts in mineral ratios and the Liver's production of Cp...

Know that the body does respond to proper nutritional inputs and sufficient time to rebuild tissue...

It's also important to know that Histamines and Methyl groups COMPETE with each other!...

That's another important factoid...

It begins to reach the realm of disbelief -- I get it...

The immune system is TOTALLY DEPENDENT on the optimal balance of Copper and Zinc, and clearly other key minerals, like Iron, Manganese to name only a few... But as you study the Anti-Oxidant Enzymes that are ESSENTIAL for Macrophage BURST, they are one of our FOUNDATIONAL 1st-line responses to neutralizing the bio-critters and pathogens!...

It is a MINERAL-Driven process to Neutralize their ascendancy and a MINERAL-Driven process to seek to overcome their presence in our bodies...

And before you take the "D"ive with all those tests, I would strongly encourage you to explore

http://allergytx.com

You are NOT broken... Allergies are NOT what your doctor says they are...

You do have "error messages" in your "Bar Code Reader" that's interpreting your environment... And what causes errors?... "Stress!"

AllergyTX is swift, painless, fascinating and a whole lot LESS expensive than conventional allergy Tx... (By the way, I have personally used this technology, I have NO interest in it, and I have referred scores of clients with great success across the country...)

Last licks, please know that Ceruloplasmin level is what REGULATES Histamine:

http://www.ncbi.nlm.nih.gov/pubmed/4630290

(The fact that there's NO Abstract suggests that this is UBER important!!!)

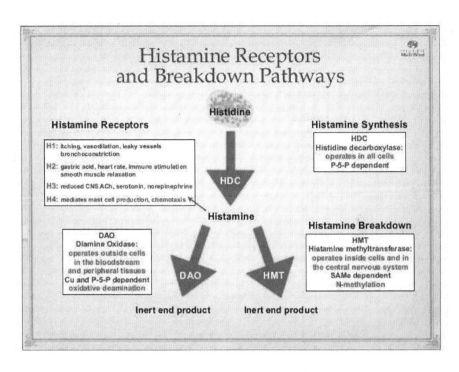

Histamine Receptors and Breakdown Pathways

Histidine

Histamine Receptors

H1: Itching, vasodilation, leaky vessels bronchoconstriction

H2: gastric acid, heart rate, immune stimulation smooth muscle relaxation

H3: reduced CNS ACh, serotonin, norepinephrine

H4: mediates mast cell production, chemotaxis

Histamine Synthesis

HDC
Histidine decarboxylase: operates in all cells
P-5-P dependent

HDC

Histamine

DAO
Diamine Oxidase: operates outside cells in the bloodstream and peripheral tissues
Cu and P-5-P dependent oxidative deamination

Histamine Breakdown

HMT
Histamine methyltransferase: operates inside cells and in the central nervous system
SAMe dependent
N-methylation

DAO

HMT

Inert end product   Inert end product

HORMONES

A slight editorial twist: Balance Minerals >> which enables Hormones to balance >> which enables Cycles to normalize... Mildred S. Seelig, MD, the greatest Mag Guru of her day, referred to Maggie as the "mineral of motion..." There is NO MORE graphic image of "motion" than in a cycling woman's body...

BCP's (birth control pills) CAUSE BOTH depletion of Mg AND build-up of unbound Copper -- a VERY BAD COMBO for our bodies!

Conventional medicine goes to GREAT L-E-N-G-T-H-S to convince you that Hormones RUN the body...

Hormone is a Greek word that means: "messenger!"

They MOVE Minerals is a MAJOR way, but the minerals come FIRST... as they ALWAYS have since time began...

Keep in mind that there's a study to prove EVERY nuance, point, and counter-point on EVERY issue in nutrition...

I would encourage you to study carefully the long-term effects of Bio-identical Hormones...

That said, please know that I am an HRT Luddite...

I strongly believe that we were designed to MAKE Hormones, NOT eat them...

Address the mineral co-factors that are ESSENTIAL to make the enzymes work that are intended to make the Hormones naturally...

In my humble opinion, it is pure Allopathetic Witchcraft that we NEED these...

There are situations, however, where they serve a critical short-term function, but to suggest use of these synthetic chemicals for the long haul is a MAJOR *tilt!*, for me...

But then I'm weird that way...

Let me come at it a bit backwardly...

If I wanted to ENSURE LOW Hormone function this is what I would do:

1)   Take steps to GUARANTEE Adrenal Dysfunction:

   a)   Pump you full of SIN-Thyroid which disrupts Adrenal function;

   b)   Push Ascorbic Acid to thwart your Iron metabolism;

   c)   Push Ferritin to ridiculous heights; and

   d)   Keep the minerals ridiculously LOW, especially Mg, Copper, and Potassium.

2)   Takes steps to KEEP Copper and Iron Dysregulated by NEVER telling you that Iron is the "D"ummy and Copper is the Ventriloquist in the Human Body... Said another way, Iron is TOTALLY dependent on OPTIMAL Copper/Ceruloplasmin status to ensure optimal metabolic function. It is worth noting the CENTRAL role for Copper and STRUCTURAL role for Iron in the synthesis of Cytochrome P-450 Enzymes -- the BACKBONE for ALL steroid hormones!...

3)   Takes steps to KEEP your Ceruloplasmin at LOW
     LEVELS by

     a)   Keeping you "Stressed Out!",

     b)   Keep Mg LOW and thus cortisol HIGH,

     c)   Pump you FULL of Hormone-D,

     d)   Terrify you about taking Retinol, among a dozen
             other steps...

4)   CONVINCE you that a LOW-FAT Diet is the Bee's
     Knees! And that Industrial Oils -- full of inflammatory-
     inducing Om-6's -- are "just" what you need...

Said another way, Healthy Adrenals and Liver are PRE-
REQUISITES for making Hormones.

You need lots of REAL Fat that delivers Fat Soluble Vitamins --
WHICH ARE **NOT** FOUND IN COCONUT OIL and OLIVE OIL --
sorry;

Optimal levels of minerals, especially Mg and Copper, and
healthy levels of Ceruloplasmin to ENSURE the Iron behaves
properly...

You also need to bring your emotional triggers and "Stressors!"
under control via EFT, Heart Math, Yoga, Exercise, etc.

Now, please study this nutrient table inspired by Shawnese
Boynton

http://nutritiondata.self.com/facts/custom/2193874/0

Indeed, Maca Root powder has been used for millennia by many
civilizations to provide the minerals and vitamins ESSENTIAL for

optimal hormone regulation by nourishing the Adrenals and Liver with what they need to work...

I would guess that MANY who've failed at "natural" hormone balancing were LOST in Steps #1-4 noted ^^^^ and actually believed what their practitioners and/or pundits were preaching...

Needed for ALL those Hormone conversions noted ^^^^:

o   Vitamin A (MIA in those LOST In "D"ementia...)

o   Bioavailable Copper and it's Ceruloplasmin powerhouse partner...

o   Maggie, easily LOST to "Stressors!" like SIN-Thyroid!...

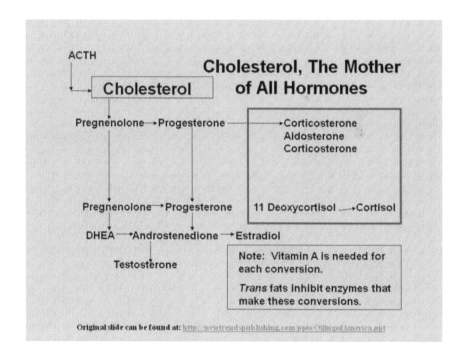

MISLED AND MISFED

Braggin about Maggie has the transcript of the podcast, for your convenience to review in detail.

Please know, I worked in Hospitals (as an exec/consultant for 32 years) thinking that you and your physician colleagues knew what you were doing...

Turns out I was wrong, and so are you and your colleagues...

And while I thump your nose, I know it's the scripted medical education and training that you received that is hopelessly twisted, "D"istorted, and for the most part, BACKWARDS. The scale of it is mind-numbing, as you are taught to RECOGNIZE "enzyme deficiency" and IGNORE the missing minerals, which ACTIVATE those enzymes, which are LOST to relentless, chronic "Stress!" -- Much of which is triggered by toxic, synthetic Rx meds, that you and your colleagues administer without questioning their mineral impact...

Hmmmmm...

So, if you wish to evolve as a practitioner, I would advise you to read WAAAAAAY more on this group BEFORE dropping into your "trained" responses about "do THIS," and do "THAT!"...

Trust me, you're not the 1st to learn you wasted 10-12 years of your life memorizing "backward" physiology, courtesy of your BIG Pharma benefactors that NOW fund and essentially OWN Medical Schools...

I'm am forever entertained by the number of folks who will put up with the ignorance and arrogance of doctors just so that they can save a few $$$$ to have the doctor order the tests that they want, even though 80+% of the time they order the WRONG tests, and then challenge them on how to interpret the results...

I encourage all my clients who will listen to step OFF the grid of convention and take control of their health STARTING with the ordering of the correct health tests and leave the hassle factor out of it...

To each their own...

http://articles.mercola.com/sites/articles/archive/2015/05/24/medical-fraud-doctoring-data.aspx

We're all busy, it's the weekend, summer's just gettin' started... I know, I know... but this is an important use of your time, and a key resource for your better understanding of the game of conventional medicine.

Please take the 21 minutes, to listen to this excerpt of Joseph Mercola, DO's interview with Malcolm Kendrick, MD, who is an impeccable clinician from Scotland, respected and outspoken critic of the "Cholesterol Con" that has held the world hostage for the last 60 years.

Dr Kendrick has just published an important new book that challenges our perception of medical research, and how wildly deceiving and flawed it can be and is, all too often.

This is an excellent expose on the so-called "science" of medicine. It is a must read for anyone really committed to gaining health independence, and knowing how challenged and distorted the "facts" of medicine really can be... This is an important work to enhance your critical thinking skills about the reality of healing...

If you're inspired by the interview, I'd strongly recommend you buy his book re same:

http://www.amazon.com/Doctoring-Data-medical-advice-nonsense-ebook/dp/B00TCG3X4S

Read this page carefully. No real benefit of Storage D over 20. Isolated D negatively impacts Mg and potassium....

http://my-Magnesium.com/hormone-d.html

Here's the "D"eal, folks...

There is a MAJOR "D"ifference between "The STORY" and "The TRUTH"...

So those seeking MORE TRUTH about Hormone-D, you might enjoy the works of:

o   Fred A. Kummerow, PhD (100-yr old Professor of Biology at U of Ill who is STILL spending 20 hours/week researching and writing!...)

o   Rick Malter, PhD (who almost killed himself with "The STORY" re the "D"eceptive Hormone)

o   Sam Queen, CCN who has distilled many of Dr. Kummerow's articles on the "D"angers of Hormone-D... This is the stuff that makes one's toes curl...

o   David L. Watts, DC, PhD who heads up TEI, and has a firm grasp on the mineral TRUTH of the human body, has written an excellent article on "Vitamin-D"... (Not for the faint of heart...)

o   Shane Ellison, MS who has written several articles on
        the absurdity of Vitamin-D supplementation

o   Todd Becker is a health writer that has written a wonderful
        piece on why he "D"oesn't supplement with "D" anymore...

o   Brian Walsh at Precision Nutrition has also spoken out
        about cautions on supplemental "D"...

Others that I'd put in the "Softly Cautioning, but Afraid to Take a
StanD against MSM's stance on this TOXIN" are the following...

(Please know, I have GREAT respect for much of their writings
and positions, but their equivocation on this topic stirs my
MBR...)

o   Suzy Cohen, RPh...
o   Carolyn Dean, MD, ND...
o   Chris Masterjohn, PhD...
o   Chris Kresser, LAc

So, there you have it... those are my "D"ream Team for
Hormone-D Contrarians... And if I've missed any obvious and
outspoken practitioners/writers, please bring them to my
attention...

Mark my words, within our lifetime, there WILL be a
WHOLESALE reversal on this issue... my greatest concern is
that it may come TOO LATE for the masses...

The window on "Homo Normalus" is closely rapidly ALL around
the Globe... and MOST are too lost in "The STORY" to see the
forest for the trees..." Sometimes, it's a bit "D"epressing...

A summer of sunshine will elevate MIGHTILY your innate Hormone-D levels... And if you're NOT consuming sufficient quantities of Retinol, animal-based Vitamin-A, it will have the SAME effect of lowering the production of Ceruloplasmin in the Liver, thereby lowering your level of Bioavailable Copper, thereby lowering your levels of anti-oxidant enzymes (SOD, and CAT, especially) and thereby INCREASING your hair loss due to the increased Oxidative Stress!...

I would advise this blood test to cut to the chase of your seasonal allopecia:
http://requestatest.com/mag-zinc-copper-panel-with-iron-panel-testing

To what extent can the Obsession over Hormone-D affect the status and function of Retinoic Acid:
http://www.sciencedirect.com/science/article/pii/S088875431100 1583

We will NOT change this dysfunctional system...

We WILL change the # of people who believe in it and are willing to RISK THEIR LIVES with it...

A General CHOOSES his/her battle... and that's MINE!...

o   The Sun "Oxidizes" things, especially our skin...

o   The MASTER Anti-oxidant enzymes are CuZnSOD, and Cerulpolasmin, both of which are Cu-dependent...

o   Anti-biotics BIND Copper...

OXALATES

This is WHY your Oxalate issue was such a problem:

http://www.ncbi.nlm.nih.gov/m/pubmed/10840464/

Avoiding High Oxalate foods makes sense in the short-term...

In the long-term, you want to up your production of SOD and CAT - BOTH of which require bioavailable Copper that can ONLY occur when the Liver is able to make Ceruloplasmin...

Said another way, it's reasonable to assume that anyone with Oxalate issues also has LOW bioavailable Copper and Ceruloplasmin...

My thinking continues to evolve re "Oxalates..."

I have NEVER bought the "endogenous producer" concept that is so popular.

Recently, I read that Oxalates "chelate" Iron...

My focus is NOW on assessing whether THAT scourge, along with Salicylates, Histamines, Amines, etc. aren't just a body ADAPTING to a toxic level of Iron and a lack of sufficient Ceruloplasmin to metabolize it...

I've shared it with select few in this "O"-world (Oxalate-world) and they're NOT on board with it. What I can also say is that those with this issue will STILL need to be careful with the wholefood form of Vit-C...

This is definitely a "work in process," but I"m breaking with convention at the present time...

OXIDATIVE STRESS

Endolymphatic Hydrops is affected by Oxidative Stress:

http://www.ncbi.nlm.nih.gov/pubmed/15811695

Caspace-3, tied with Oxidative Stress, is triggered by Copper deficiency:

http://www.ncbi.nlm.nih.gov/pubmed/14608045

Trust me, the intersection of Mg deficiency and Copper dysregulation is at the CORE of this dynamic -- AND MOST CHRONIC DISEASE -- although that's NOT what your doctor believes...

As difficult as it is to believe, there is NO such thing as Medical Disease...

There is, however, OVERWHELMING evidence that Mineral Deficiencies CAUSE Metabolic Dysfunction...
Focus on the production of Ceruloplasmin -- please do NOT obsess about your Copper status...

Oxidative stress in women....

This article may shed some light on the origin of your fibroids:
http://journals.plos.org/plosone/article?id=10.1371%2Fjournal.pone.0072069

Oxidative Stress is the intersection of LOW Anti-Oxidant Enzymes, and excess, unbound Copper and Iron. And, there's likely some heavy metal dynamics in the thick of this, as well...

EAT IT, OR DRINK IT??

Smoothies how do you all neutralize the mineral blocking effect of Phytates in RAW food?!?...

Our bodies are made to chew to digest, no chew creates chaos!?!

SILICA AND ALUMINUM

Silica to reduce aluminum in HTMA.......

Fiji Water that has high amounts of Silica... Also, I've had MANY clients clear their Aluminum with sustained and proper supplementation with Maggie...

Invariably what happens, however, is that Hair levels of Calcium will SHOOT UP, and then calm down in subsequent HTMAs...

Also note that Aluminum WHIPS up Iron in a wicked way... In fact, I think that's one reason WHY it's sooooo prevalent in our environment...

http://www.ncbi.nlm.nih.gov/pubmed/?term=Magnesium%20177%25%20silica

CONDITIONS

ALCOHOLISM

I ain't no "tea-totaller," but I grew up in a family that "loved" its alcohol...

If someone had told them that there was a SERIOUS price to be paid for that habit (Mg Lossand Iron retention in their Liver), and that the obsession for alcohol was driven by both Mg and Copper deficiency, then things might have turned out differently...

And the researcher that we should thank for this insight is Edmund B. Flink, MD, PhD... He figured it out!

http://www.ncbi.nlm.nih.gov/pubmed/3544909

ALZHEIMERS (AD)

AD is CAUSED by Cu deficiency at birth and this affects structure and development of Hippocampus. Lack of Cu reduces Cu,Zn-SOD and allows build-up of Aluminum that THEN depletes Maggie... I've NO idea where Sodium and Boron are in that mineral dance...

Let's keep one thing straight...

o   Ceruloplasmin "activates" Copper (and Iron, for that matter...)

o   Metallothionein "stores" Copper...

There is a MAJOR difference in their metabolic function and purpose INSIDE the body...

And when it comes to the KEY metals, they are actually a quadrant:

o   Copper
o   Zinc
o   Iron
o   Manganese

And with the exception of Zinc, all the others have a metabolic NEED and relationship with Ceruloplasmin...

Zinc BLOCKS Copper absorption... Zn/Cu is a MAJOR seesaw in the body...

Please ignore the reference in this article to Parkinson's... The underlying concepts are IDENTICAL for Alzheimer's:

http://www.hindawi.com/journals/omcl/2014/147251/

http://www.ncbi.nlm.nih.gov/m/pubmed/22708607/

Lack of Ceruloplasmin (Cp) appears to be the more relevant FALL guy...

Once again, ALL is not as it seems...

Please know that anyone dealing with the condition of Alzheimer's has a notable imbalance in their Copper and Iron, which would support the notion that these metals are instrumental in the dynamics of Alzheimer's. This is noted in these abstracts and several other articles that are noted below:

http://articles.mercola.com/sites/articles/archive/2013/09/12/copper-alzheimers-disease.aspx

http://www.sciencedirect.com/science/article/pii/S0022510X98000926

http://www.medicalnewstoday.com/articles/265012.php

This 3rd article comes the closest to explaining the overview of this dynamic...

The build-up of bio-unavailable Copper CREATES metabolic DEFICIENCY of Copper and a shortage of critical Copper proteins that are ESSENTIAL for optimal brain function.

I can assure you, it is a rare physician who has ANY knowledge of these mineral deficiencies and the extent to which they create the metabolic dysfunctions that lead to a constellation of symptoms known as Alzheimer's... In my humble opinion, it is NOT a disease! It is a gross dysregulation of minerals.

The inability of the Copper dysregulated body to produce sufficient anti-oxidant enzymes, esp. SOD, CAT and GSH, is at the core of this dynamic that is shrouded in mystery and mineral denialism.

https://www.facebook.com/groups/MagnesiumAdvocacy/923175287750541/

https://www.facebook.com/groups/MagnesiumAdvocacy/923175997750470/

https://www.facebook.com/groups/MagnesiumAdvocacy/923176464417090/

https://www.facebook.com/groups/MagnesiumAdvocacy/923176647750405/

https://www.facebook.com/groups/MagnesiumAdvocacy/923176647750405/

https://www.facebook.com/groups/MagnesiumAdvocacy/923176917750378/

https://www.facebook.com/groups/MagnesiumAdvocacy/923177044417032/

https://www.facebook.com/groups/MagnesiumAdvocacy/923177107750359/

ANESTHESIA

What sort of Anesthesia was used for the surgery?... If it was a general, it is most likely activated with Fluoride, which has a notable effect on your mineral status, especially Maggie...

That would be the 1st on my list of things to check on...

And you might note the tightening of the doctor's sphincters when you ask about this little discussed "D"own-side of surgery...

ANXIETY / PANIC ATTACKS

Please read:

http://drhoffman.com/article/panic-attacks-and-anxiety-2/

ALL forms of Maggie will enable Thiamine, Vit-B1, to work properly and restore the much needed Mg lost to "Stress!" and the perception of threat...

There is NO one form of Mg that works for all...

And the form that you are recommending is very popular, but does LITTLE to restore Mg status... it tops off, but it does not replenish cellular stores...

So can Mag Help?

In a word, Yes!

In a lot of words, this explains WHY:

http://www.ncbi.nlm.nih.gov/m/pubmed/21835188/

Dosing of Magnesium = (5mgs Maggie/lb or 10mgs/kg)

Given that panic attacks are the intersection of Mg deficiency and Copper dysregulation, I'm not clear how this product moves the needle?...

75mg of Mg a day is pathetic, Ascorbic Acid does NOT solve the Copper<>Cp dynamic and synthetic B's do NOT rebuild tissue.

They "stimulate," but they do NOT restore the metabolic deficiency...

I'm hesitant, it beats Xanax, but this approach doesn't seem to be going far enough...

ATHSMA

Sarah Myhill, MD uses MgCl oil in nebulizers to address the symptoms of "Athsma" naturally...

http://drmyhill.co.uk/wiki/Magnesium_-_treating_a_deficiency

15 parts Distilled Water
1part MgCl oil
Breathe...

AVASCULAR NECROSIS

Avascular Necrosis of the hip.

Looks like the culprit is Oxidative Stress:

http://medicine-hygiene.idnwhois.org/article-189837.html

I'd be focusing on production of Ceruloplasmin (Cp) to ensure bioavailable Cu to run the Anti-Oxidant enzymes, and reduce bio-unavailable Fe to PREVENT oxidative "Stress!".

If you've been engaged with Hormone-D, it has likely overwhelmed your Liver Vit-A status and seriously affected Ceruloplasmin (Cp) production...

BED WETTING

It's a Histamine reaction...

It is affected by LOW Mg, Cu and B6...

Healthy Copper levels... The more relevant factor is to address Ceruloplasmin, the protein that makes Copper "usable." This protein needs to be ~35md/dL...

Most people are <20!

THAT lack of sufficent Cp to run our bodies is the true Stealth Health issue -- worldwide!...

BESTOW A BEATING HEART

Please know that MOST, if not ALL, Rx meds for the heart have warnings...

So, let me connect the dots...

o   Hearts with symptoms lack sufficient energy to keep the heart going 24/7... (It's the ONLY muscle in our bodies that NEVER rests...)

o   Energy is spelled Mg-ATP INSIDE the cells, and especially INSIDE the Heart's cells (aka, cardiomyocytes)...

o   Many Cardiac Rx meds CAUSE Hypomagnesemia... (That means that Mg's SOOOO LOW that it shows LOW on a SERUM blood test!...)

o   Who does THIS ^^^ make sense to?!?...

What differences in the Heart Beat REALLY mean...

o   Pounding Heart Beat => TOO MUCH Calcium... (from a lack of Mg)

o   Racing Heart Beat => TOO MUCH Sodium... (from excess Iron in the Heart that CAUSES a LOSS of Maggie and then Potassium, and a RISE in Sodium due to the lack of Mg and K...)

o   Irregular Heart Beat => TOO LITTLE Potassium... (most likely from TOO MUCH synthetic Hormone-D, because the "Vitamin-D blood test showed LOW, but it was ACTUALLY from TOO LITTLE Maggie" and Iron has a wicked effect on Potassium status, as well...)

Contrary to popular or medical opinion, ALL Heart issues come back to Magnesium status... and what I am learning with increasing facility and fervor is that Iron Overload (excess, mismanaged Iron due to a lack of Ceruloplasmin...) is at the BASE OF ALL THIS METABOLIC INSANITY...

BLOODY NOSES

My $$$'s on fragile capillaries due to insufficient Lysyl Oxidase enzyme which is what gives tissue, especially blood vessels, arteries and capillaries sufficient strength and flexibility. The enzyme that ensures tissue integrity is Lysyl Oxidase -- that enzyme is Copper dependent.

The easiest way to increase the uptake of Copper is using Wholefood Vit-C -- NOT Ascorbic Acid. Good brands are: Innate Response, Grown by Nature, Garden of Eden, Pure Radiance, SP Cataplex C are among the leaders. Likely you will need at least the RDA of WF Vit-C of 60mgs/day.

Noting all the above, are there any Copper related issues that seem to run in the family?...

BLOOD SUGAR

Please read "30-Day Diabetes Cure" and spend some time on www.bloodsugar101.com.

Yes, Type 1Diabetes is a different beast than T2D. Based on my research, it's a combination of Zinc and Mg that make the biggest difference in your demand for Insulin. And and excess storage of Iron in the pancreas has a chilling impact on BOTH!...

It would likely be wise to get the following blood tests to assess what's really going on:

o   Mag RBC
o   Plasma Zinc
o   Serum Copper
o   Serum Ceruloplasmin
o   A1c
o   Fasting Blood Glucose
o   Serum Iron
o   Serum Transferrin
o   Serum TIBC (% SAT)
o   Serum Ferritin

BRUISING

Capillary fragility is what causes "bruising," at least as best I understand it...

Bio-available Copper (properly bound to its transport protein, Ceruloplasmin), working with wholefood Vit-C complex, is what is KEY to good collagen formation that enables proper creation of blood vessel walls...

It is an early, and easily overlooked form of Scurvy.

And we ALL know that Wholefood Vitamin C is the solution to THAT problem. (It just requires using the CORRECT form of Vitamin-C, OK?)

CANDIDA

This is a bit dry, but I think begins to pull back the curtain on some key metabolic dynamics that affect susceptibility to Candida:

http://jid.oxfordjournals.org/content/175/6/1467.long

There is GREAT confusion in conventional circles to OBSESS over Iron and IGNORE Copper status... And I believe FAR TOO MANY folks supplement with Iron, when, IN FACT, their so-called "anemia" is CAUSED by a lack of bioavailable Copper...

So here's my theory:

"Stress!" >> Mg Loss >> Rise of Stress Hormones >> Lack of Cp production in the Liver >> Rise of unbound Copper/Fall of bound Copper >> Fall of Anti-Oxidant Enzymes >> Rise of unbound Iron (it needs Cp, too!) >> Rise of Oxidative Stress (due to Increased Iron and decreased Enzymes) >> Rise of Candida...

I believe the mineral imbalance and metabolic assault comes FIRST, and the opportunistic pathogen FOLLOWS...

Iron Overload Alters Innate and T-Helper Cell Responses to Candida albicans in Mice

http://jid.oxfordjournals.org/content/175/6/1467.long

Let's start with lowering that "Stress!" and apply the recommended protocol within that context... As the level of bioavailable Copper rises (with the increased Cp), yes, the body should come into better balance.

And remember, EFT is a wonderful resource to "reset" our response to "Stress!"

Let's be sure to keep one thing in mind re Copper and ATP...

MOST who are sucking wind re "proper" Copper are chronically "Stressed Out!" and their Livers lack the natural mojo to make Ceruloplasmin (Cp), a KEY antioxidant enzyme of its own right...

This coupled with the fact that "Stress!" DEPLETES Mg -- it's how we're wired as a species. And ATP without Mg DOES NOT WORK. ATP MUST have that mineral:

1) To change its stereochemical structure...

2) To change its valence (-4 >> -2)

3) To change its viability inside the cell...

In my world, Maggie and proper Copper are the Conductor (Mg) and 1st Violin (Cu) of the Cellular Orchestra of minerals INSIDE our cells...

They are BOTH essential to make beautiful music, and note that a violinist is LOST without her/his bow (Cp)...

Please know that E-SOD (Red Blood Cell), and L-SOD (White blood cell) are KEY to keeping Yeast in check... And yes, Copper is ESSENTIAL to make them both of them function...

Who knew?...

CELIAC

I don't believe it's "celiac/gluten sensitivity..."

I do believe it is "Glyphosate Toxicity..."

Let's be clear about what we're REALLY reacting to...

It AIN'T the wheat that's the problem... It's what they're spraying on it BEFORE they harvestist...

Glyphosate is the fancy name for RoundUp!...

It is BOTH a mineral chelator and an anti-biotic... (Primary targets for this chemical are COPPER and Magnesium...)

It is toxic to our mineral health, and thus our overall health... And I certainly believe Monsanto when it says it "doesn't do this in Europe..." Right!...

http://www.americanradioworks.publicradio.org.../global.html

Genes ONLY express when the EPIGENETIC STRESSORS stimulate them...

The "Germ" Theory AND "Gene" Theory are TOTAL BS, in my humble opinion!!!!

A celiac's "environment" ain't strong enough or balanced enough, yet. And yes, TOTAL lack of GMO (Glyphosate) is KEY to gaining proper balance...

***Also, refer to the Copper and Glyphosate Chapter!

CYSTIC FIBROSIS

A starting point would be to pursue WHY you have cystic fibrosis. This article certainly sheds important light on that issue:

http://www.ncbi.nlm.nih.gov/pubmed/14681839

Know that the metabolic activities of Fat REQUIRE optimal Copper stores and properly bound Copper...

Instead of chasing the Paper Tiger of her LOW Storage-D (which ONLY means that you're Magnesium Deficient... please re-read that sentence again... ^^^^), I would be doing these two sets of tests to get to the TRUTH:

o http://requestatest.com/mag-zinc-copper-panel-with-iron-panel-testing

o https://requestatest.com/mag-vitamin-d-panel--testing

(Please know to eliminate the duplicate Mag RBC...)

That's where I'd START to focus...

Please know that lack of bioavailable Copper creates the ILLUSION of a "genetic" issue, when in fact this is a "generational" issue that has been building for the last 4-5 generations due to the rampant dysregulation of Copper by the agricultural, food and pharmaceutical industries...

Forgive me, I don't mean to come off as a "genetic luddite..." I'm just seeking to shed light on OTHER aspects of these dynamics likely not covered in your research.

ALL is NOT as it seems... The VAST majority of so-called genetic conditions are triggered by epi-genetic "Stress!"

My youngest daughter has Down Syndrome... Know that I'm not a casual researcher about this dynamic...

Your Mineral Denialist's understanding of Calcitriol metabolism is pedestrian, at best, in my humble opinion.

And what is their Mag RBC? Hormone-D testing without KNOWING Intracellular Magnesium is very risky and irrelevant...

Totally understand that...

MAG is NOT unlike The Wizard of Oz, where we'll teach you that the "Wizard" is, IN FACT, a snake oil salesman, and we'll ALSO teach you how to use those Ruby Slippers so you can take back control of your health...

DEPRESSION

Best way to "prevent" depression is manage the ratio of Calcium/Magnesium. This has been known for a long, long time:

http://qjmed.oxfordjournals.org/content/os-24/95/371.extract

Now, there are three sisters that run together in the body:

Calcium, Copper and Estrogen.

Many of my female clients took BCPs for some period of time, thereby flooding their bodies with Estrogen, and as a result have high levels of Calcium and excess, hidden, unbound Copper due to lack of ceruloplasmin...

And those same women were never told that Maggie is the anti-dote to all three: Mg is nature's Calcium antagonist and regulator; Mg when attached to Mg-ATP allows Copper to bind to Ceruloplasmin so it can be properly used; and Mg activates key enzymes in the Liver to enhance their removal and activate other key enzymes that get the Estrogen Receptors to work properly again.

Remember, Hormones are "messengers." When their "Cellphones" (receptors) don't work properly, they can't communicate with each other, and especially with the Hypothalamus -- BIG problem. Again, I realize I'm a dog with a bone, but minerals are the agents for balance and mood leveling. They ensure symmetry, and when out of balance, the body kicks in Neurotransmitters and Hormones for swift corrective action... And flip Copper from bioavailable to bioUNavailable and you'll tweak TWO KEY enzymes:

o   GAD (glutamic acid decarboxylase)
o   DBM (Dopamine beta-monooxygenase)

And when THAT happens, DEPRESSION follows..

It is BIOLOGICAL -- NOT GENETIC!...

The "feelings" being assessed in EPDS are a function of mineral levels and ratios and the consequent impact on the function of KEY enzymes that produce hormones and Neurotransmitters... This is NOT Rocket Science -- regrettably, this is BASIC biology that ALL deserve to know and MASTER...

EHLER DANLOS SYNDROME (EDS)

Ehler Danlos Syndrome is "billed" as genetic, but MAG me with a spoon:

https://rarediseases.org/rare-diseases/ehlers-danlos-syndrome/

Make Copper dysfunctional and NOT bioavailable, and Lysyl Oxidase will NOT work!... This is an ENTIRELY Copper dependent enzyme.

It is NOT "genetic," but it is "generational" due to the vacuous state of minerals in the womb of the last 3-4 generations of women...

Ehlors Danlos syndrome as I understand EDS (which is arguably limited...)

It is HIGHLY correlated with under-functioning of Lysyl Oxidase, which is a VITAL enzyme that ensures blood vessel and tissue integrity, strength and flexibility -- not an insignificant set of factors for healthy bodies.

Lack of bioavailable Copper, for a WIDE variety of factors, would certainly be a complicating factor.

And how does Copper go South?!?... With the rise of "Stress!"

Hormones from too much loss of Maggie, the Liver slows/stops its production of Ceruloplasmin (Cp) which sends Copper into a tail-spin...

FOOD ALLERGIES

Please also refer to Histamines.

I would encourange you to explore: (there is also a website in Australia...)

http://allergytx.com

I've personally used this technology and can attest to its effectiveness and staying power... I've had scores of clients benefit from it, as well...

Food intolerances are merely another "Stressor!" that CAUSES mineral imbalance, and Magnesium LOSS...

"Stress!" >> Electrolyte Derangement >> Energy (Mg-ATP) LOSS >> Inflammation >> Fibrosis

I don't entirely know where, but "auto-immune" is a part of the dynamic of Energy Loss >> Inflammation. The body attacking itself is a classic "Stress!" Response -- it is NOT a "disease..."

Food intolerances are often "error messages" going to the brain. An option here in the States and in Australia is outlined in the above website.

This stops the vicious cycle. There are variations of this approach that can be used to address this issue, stem the loss of nutrients, and start the process to restore and re-balance the minerals...

GALL BLADDER

High bilirubin is the offending agent of Gall Bladders, especially when they get OXIDIZED due to too little anti-oxidant enzymes for LACK OF BIOAVAILABLE Copper...

Do the Liver/Gall Bladder Flush... Avoid the ravages of surgery... I personally have done this -- more than 20 years ago -- and have recommended this approach to dozens of colleagues, friends and family members...

http://www.fitfoodhouse.net/completely-natural-and-easy-way-to-remove-gallstones-its-good-for-your-liver-too/

I have "free" pizza's for LIFE (not that I would eat them...) from a Pizza Mogul in Chicago who avoided surgery by my simply suggesting he do a Liver/Gall Bladder flush before his scheduled surgery...

The long-term implications of "removing" that VITAL organ are STAGGERING!... (Despite the assurances of your scalpel wielding surgeon...)

HAIR LOSS - ALLOPECIA

From what I am piecing together, ALL auto-immune diseases are CAUSED by Copper deficiency... Allopecia (hair loss) is considered another form of auto-immune condition.

I would focus stemming her optimizing Copper bioavailability. Another issue, are the B-Vitamins. You might try Nutritional Yeast (NO, it won't cause a Candida infection...) as it is a great source of the yeast that MAKE the B's and has Copper in it, as well...

As for the ACV(Apple Cider Vinegar), it's a very rich source of Potassium that has a dynamic relationship with both Maggie and Copper and Iron!...

And the beat goes on...

To the point, there are multiple factors that are associated with Hair Loss and Hair Recovery, but at the end of the trail, it is a common set of mineral factors that dictate optimal metabolism and hair health... not the least of which is our "sponsor," Maggie!

Please also refer to Balancing Hormones.

HYPOKALEMIA

Here's an Excellent article on this issue:

http://jasn.asnjournals.org/content/18/10/2649.full

Bottom line: Mg rules the Electrolytes. Period.

From what I understand, and it is explored in this article... You cannot restore Potassium levels until Mg is replete. And what precedes ALL Potassium loss is Mg loss... And where does this happen frequently?...

With Rx meds designed to lower BP, ALL of which cause massive losses of Mg AND Potassium. And doctors ignore the Mg issue and suggest Potassium tablets at 99mgs, despite the daily requirement being ~4,700mgs of Potassium daily.

HYPERPARATHYROIDISM

Hyperparathyroidism and proper mineral replacement, please read this entire article:

http://www.tandfonline.com/.../10.../07315724.2009.10719764

ALL facets of Calcium metabolism are REGULATED by Magnesium status: PTH, Calcitonin and Hormone-D...
You might also read:

http://www.mgwater.com/gacontro.shtml

Please check your Mag RBC for starters...

Based on my reading and reflection of the research on hyperparathyroidisn is the abject ignorance re Mg's control role in regulating these nodules on the BACK of the THYROID.

The tragedy is that the REASON your Parathyroid acted out is due to LOW Magnesium status -- and that's a fact! It AIN'T no disease...

This is the panel that I've had increasing success with using:

http://requestatest.com/mag-zinc-copper-panel-with-iron-panel-testing

I would strongly advise you to lower your expectations that your Endo will:

1)   Agree to order these Metabolically REVEALING mineral tests

2)   Have a clue how to properly interpret them BEYOND whether they are "within the lines or not..."

And at the risk of seeming like an HTMA Pimp, I would also recommend an HTMA to assess your overall mineral profile to better understand your "Stress!" Profile and your ability to generate Energy in light of that "Stress!"

http://gotmag.org/work-with-us/

IBS

Safest route to take for folks with gut issues is Mg Cl oil or related approaches to bypass the tummy...

IBS and mag absorption. This'll keep you away from the Telly or out of the Pubs for a couple of hours...

http://www.ncbi.nlm.nih.gov/pmc/articles/PMC3781198/

Please note that the potency of the anti-oxidant enzyme system is DEPENDENT on the bioavailability of Copper and the LACK of excess, unmanaged Iron...

INFLAMMATION

I just want folks to KNOW Inflammation is NOT a Medical Disease...

It is a natural metabolic process to remove cells that are dying for lack of energy (ATP) that REQUIRE Minerals (especially Mg and Copper) to produce... The key is to determine WHY the minerals are in a state of loss ("Stress!") and deficiency ("Oxidative Stress!")...

Lower the "Stressors!" and FEED the cellular starvation...

Here is a key article to explain the fact that Inflammation is CAUSE by Mg deficiency:

URL: http://www.ncbi.nlm.nih.gov/pubmed/1384353

KIDNEY STONES

If the issue is "Stones," then you've got to be thinking about a LACK of Magnesium and B6...

And low and behold, THAT'S EXACTLY what causes "Stones" to form... It is NOT a medical disease...

Anytime the Kidneys act out, I'd be pursuing Copper/Iron dysregulation...

Lack of bioavailable Copper will create a Free Radical Storm (ROS) that will result in fibrosis (calcification...)

Given that the Mg is strong, I would suspect an imbalance in the Liver's production of Ceruloplasmin (Cp) which is essential to make Both Copper and Iron usable...

MIGRAINES

Migraines are very often triggered by Histamine Intolerance, which suggests issues with Mg, B6 and Copper, as ALL 3 are needed to activate the two enzymes (DAO and HNMT) that are needed to degrade them. This could involve Maggie, but possibly...

o   Too little B6...
o   Too much UNbound Copper...
o   Too little Bound Copper... and
o   Too much stored Iron that creates an oxidizing storm that eats up Anti-Oxidant Enzymes that depend on Bound Copper for their function...

That's a lot of switch-backs, I realize, but it's likely NOT just a Mg issue...

Hope that makes sense....

I'm in total agreement about the need for regular Chiropractic adjustments, but given the range of symptoms involved, I'm inclined to say that there's notable metabolic imbalance (food sensitivities, hair loss, systemic fatigue, etc.) that's been building for a number of years...

MULTIPLE SCLEROSIS (MS)

o   A GREAT option is to try Reishi... very high in Vitamin-C
       and Copper... Hmmmmm...

o   So it appears that Copper is KEY to endorphins...

http://ajcn.nutrition.org/content/43/1/42.full.pdf+html

o   MS is an auto-immune condition, like the other 30+
       auto-immune conditions... And what is the CORE issue
       for ALL of these issues?... Lack of Bioavailable Copper
       and Iron! Without exception, the lack of sufficient
       CuZnSOD allows for a notable build-up of Oxidative
       "Stress!" which triggers the metabolic breakdown that is
       assocaited with MS...

Hmmmmmmmmm...

Anyone else connecting the dots here?!?...

MTHFR

http://www.spectracell.com/media/uploaded/1/0e2676833_13854
09127_1003methylation-wheel1113.pdf

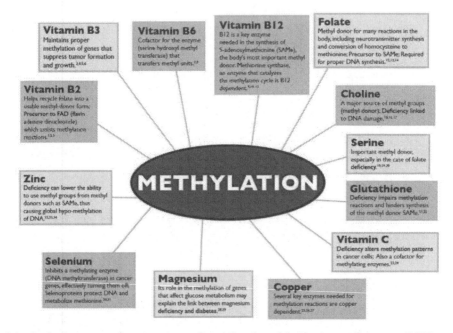

Methylation requires proper functioning Methytransferase (MT) enzymes...

Of the 10 Methyltransferase (MT) enzymes I've studied carefully (BHMT, COMT, etc.), all 10 of them REQUIRE Copper to be activated... There are 150-200 MT enzymes in the body...

In addition, please know that B-Vitamins are also known as "biogenic amines..." That means that they will NOT work until they are "oxidized" by Ceruloplasmin (Cp), a vital enzyme that requires 8 Copper atoms to work PROPERLY... (Please ignore the current literature that says Cp only needs 6 atoms..)

And what is key to the optimal stereochemical structure of Cp?...

Magnesium!....and it performs a similar role with ATP making that KEY energy chemical usable, as Mg-ATP....

Just a thought perhaps that the imbalances caused by improper supplementation might have caused a genetic expression on a snp...

Yes, that's a safe bet, given that ALL SNPs are expressions of epi-gentic (i.e. ENVIRONMENTAL) "Stressors!"... The question then remains, at what point will these transcription errors revert BACK to their original status?...

That's, in my humble opinion, is the $64 million question that is NOT adequately explored on the MTHFR research and the related websites and forums... From what I've read, these SNPs are NOT permanent, but that's the VERY impression we're left with...

Now, you're "officially" broken...

And for those that doubt this concept of reversibility of function, please familiarize yourself with Francis M. Pottenger, MD, and his infamous cats!

o http://www.biospiritual-energy-healing.com/raw-food-diet...

o http://www.amazon.com/Pottengers-CatsA.../dp/0916764060

Ask your colleagues to explain how the ENZYMES work that regulate and repair genes and gene transcription when minerals are LOST to "Stressors!" easily lost to today's food and Rx medical system...

Dr. Richard Olree is a MINERAL MEGA-STAR!...

Where most of us mortals are happy to be able to do basic arithmetic and multiplication, Dr. Olree is practicing a mathematical blend of differential equations with Calculus!... His material is MIND-BLOWING, and he's a hoot to chat with, which I've had the pleasure to do on a couple of occasions...

The metabolic switch for genes is methylation, and more specifically, Methyltransferase enzymes. There are 150-200 MT enzymes that have been identified.

I've studied 10 very closely (e.g. BHMT, COMT, HNMT, etc.) and those are ALL dependent on bioavailable Copper to work effectively. And what entered my research wheel this am was the fact that excess Iron (known as "Iron Overload" in research circles) can wreak havoc with these enzymes via its known ability to activate Hydroxyl Radicals that are legendary for damaging lipid membranes, necleotide protiens and DNA... Hmmmmmmm...

https://ntischool.com/2015/06/dr-richard-olree-on-minerals-for-the-genetic-code-part-1/

So, is Iron Overload the true, but hidden, factor behind the psycho-drama known as MTHFR?... I don't know that we can answer that question at this point, and I need to read the article ^^^^ by Dr. Olree very carefully (which I've yet to do...), but this notion that we're "genetically broken" is woefully inadequate and wrong.

For those that want to better understand how Iron creeps into our environment and our bodies, you might find this a fascinating read:

http://freetheanimal.com/2015/06/enrichment-theory-everything.html

And to further refute the "genetic vs epigenetic" origin of this dynamic, just this morning, I received this advertisement (which I'm not pumping, please...), but it does challenge the "genes are cemented in concrete" mentality of most practitioners and scientists today. Genes "driving" disease is ENTIRELY a case of "Social Construction of Reality" in the same way that "Cholesterol CAUSES Heart Disease." We know BETTER now. Enjoy this info:

http://www.howtoreprogramyourdna.com/

We have MUCH to learn about HOW our bodies get out of balance, and that, in fact, minerals play a pivotal role to bring us back to metabolic homeostasis...

It's ALL about moving those niggly little electrons around the body, right?...

ONE FOR THE LITTLE PEOPLE

It's a well-established FACT, that growth issues involve both Zinc and Copper...

More often than not, kiddo's are dealing with Copper issues given the dysfunction of Copper and Iron in the Mom's given that they are exposed to an environment "D"esigned to LOWER Copper and RAISE Iron -- which is NOT a good combination...

Thanks for the update and we'll look forward to hearing about his Ceruloplasmin (Cp) status. And just for the record, I'm MIGHTILY impressed that the doctor brought up the Cp--unaided... That's most exciting!

Breast-fed or Bottle-fed?...
Vaxx or not?...
Exposure to HFCS?...

Depending on how well you regulated the increase in Copper with the 1st pregnancy might be a compelling factor. Also, if you took Pre-Natals with excess Iron, as most have, you might have created an imbalance there...

Copper and Iron are joined at the hip of Ceruloplasmin (Cp) and if that precious protein/enzyme/anti-oxidant is dysregulated, it will affect BOTH metals...

POSTPARTUM DEPRESSION

Back-to-back pregnancies will depleted you of a significant amount of minerals... (10% for each child, and you were likely NOT @ 100% BEFORE you got pregnant -- most aren't today...)

Please read this:

http://www.ncbi.nlm.nih.gov/pmc/articles/PMC3430492/pdf/IJPS-5-40.pdf

Please get your minerals properly assessed:

o   Overall assessment, via a Hair Tissue Mineral Analysis (HTMA)

o   Targeted assessment, via the blood markers.

My hypothesis is that the combined Mg loss and Copper dysregulation have combined to affect several key enzymes that affect mood and our perception of our environment.

You are NOT losing it! Your body and mind are STARVED for proper nutrients and minerals!

Hope that helps...

 (P.S. my Dad was a manic-depressive -- I'm not a casual observer of this dynamic...)

What is HORRIBLY depressing about this thread is how "confused" and "trained" people are by what is at the FOUNDATION of this post-maternal dynamic...

Minerals ACTIVATE Enzymes! Every Enzymes that CONTROLS our mood and state of emotional balance.

Enzymes do the following:

o   Regulate the Hypothalamus...

o   Make Hormones...

o   Make Neurotransmitters...

o   Keep metabolic functions in BALANCE...

Enzymes do NOT work without Minerals... Period!

Please, I encourage one and ALL to step beyond your BIG Pharma-induced "belief system" about how the body works, and start to embrace the "biological system" that clearly demonstrates the powerful and supreme role of minerals in our health and well-being...

STOMACH ACID

Forgive me, folks... So now we're supposed to get excited that one physician recognizes the central importance of the mineral that runs the human metabolism?...

It is a start, yes I'll grant that. It comes after a CENTURY of denial and ignorance.

Here's my ACID-TEST question: "If they *missed* the most BASIC aspect of human physiology, what else are they getting wrong?!?"

I can assure you, their FAILURE re Maggie is but the TIP of an iceberg of inadequacy and incompetence...

And while I know my piercing observations make some of you uncomfortable, I can assure you that they are NOT my opinions, but ARE backed by scientific FACT, that is clearly outlined in the hundreds (~2,500 thus far) of articles that I've read on minerals and mineral metabolism...

Allopathetic Medicine is Affagato...

There are 170,000 Mineral Denialists -- in the US alone -- that are in "D"enial regarding the supremacy of minerals...

Point of reference, Burton and Bella Altura, PhD(s) have published over 1,000 scientific, peer-reviewed articles in VERY stuffy journals in their storied career re Magnesium and Mg deficiency and it's IMPACT on the human metabolism...

All any physician who is SERIOUS about healing need do is read JUST the ABSTRACTS to those 1,000+ articles...It's very clearly spelled out - for those seeking to learn the TRUTH...

Please follow the bouncing balls...

o   Proper Stomach HCl Acid requires Zinc, B1, B6 and Iodine...

o   "Stress!" CAUSES the loss of Mg, Zn and B-Vitamins...

o   A most disruptive form of stress is "Oxidative Stress!"

o   "Oxidative Stress" is intensified by Excess, Unmanaged Iron...

o   In my world, excess Iron, Iron fortification (HFCS, GMO, etc) disrupts production of HCl via its tug-of-war with Zinc..

o   Now, H.pylori LOVES an Iron-filled environment... Hmmmmmm...

o   Copper and Ceruloplasmin are ESSENTIAL to manage Iron...

o   An excellent source of Copper is Wholefood Vit-C -- NOT Ascorbic Acid...

o   Research in the 1940's clearly indicated that H.pylori was destroyed by Ascorbate + Copper (aka WF Vit-C)...

o   So, again, in my world, BOTH the Excess Iron >> H.pylori is addressed by Copper (WF Vit-C..)...

o   Address the Iron and restore the Stomach HCl Acid...

o   I wouldn't get near an Anti-biotic (NOR a PPI) if you paid
          me!!!

OK, let's agree that stomach acid requires Cl, Mg and B3 and
B6... But we seem to have THREE different perceptions of an
additional mineral:

o   Zinc (lost to "Stress!" and PPIs)

o   Copper (loses bioavailability with Stress!")

o   Calcium -- makes no sense to me...

Can anybody clarify and sort this out?!?

Rick Malter

*More than 30 years ago in their HTMA seminars in Phoenix, AZ,
Drs. Paul Eck and David Watts, knew that slow oxidizers with
very low sodium and potassium levels weren't able to produce
adequate amounts of HCL to efficiently digest food, especially
proteins.*

*They needed HCL to support digestion until their adrenals were
strengthened and their sodium and potassium levels increased.*

*This process will vary from individual to individual. You have to
be cautious about overgeneralizing when it comes to HTMA and
nutrition issues.*

*The intra cellular minerals -- magnesium (Mg) and potassium (K)
-- usually take longer to build up adequate reserves than many of
the other minerals. Also stress accelerates the Mg burn rate so
that Mg levels can drop rather quickly.*

*Copper dumping also can deplete potassium levels rather
quickly. Remember, the nutrient minerals are part of a complex*

dynamic system that needs to be monitored periodically with HTMA re-tests.

Copper toxic slow oxidizers with very low sodium and potassium levels (low HCL) usually take much more time to detox and re-balance minerals than fast oxidizers who usually don't have the HCL insufficiency.

The challenge for fast oxidizers is to reduce their stress level (high sodium level) so that they can retain more Mg and build their Mg reserves.

Another important aspect of HTMAs, and the mineral system that they reflect, is that the minerals usually relate to multiple health functions.

For example, the low sodium and potassium levels in a copper toxic slow oxidizer HTMA not only relate to low HCL production in the stomach, but also to low production of ceruloplasmin (Cp) to bind copper and make it bio-available.

An increase in adrenal strength is needed for both HCL and Cp production.

Independent MAG-Pie

Take a stomach acid pill (something with say, betaine hydrochloride as an example.. but be aware betaine is a methyl donor), if it burns it's because stomach lining thickens in response to stomach acid and thin lining will burn when you add too much acid.

If you have a zinc, B6 or Mg deficiency you've got low stomach acid as those are needed to make it.

Any protein intolerance would also indicate this (but that's not the sole cause of protein intolerance). Fats and protein cannot be broken down in an alkaline environment.

Drinking cabbage juice before a meal can promote its production, as can Swedish bitters, gentian (low sals herb) tincture, homemade saurkraut, sprinkling a little of the contents of a stomach acid supp onto the food and gradually increasing as tolerated.
If a stool test returns steathorrhea (fat malapsorption) that could be low stomach acid too, as could a positive test result of Helicobactor pylori. Once the food starts to digest properly, pathogenic bugs don't grow as much and reinfection is less likely, so dysbiosis improves. .

This is temporary until the underlying mineral imbalance is restored!

SUGAR

Braggin about Maggie has the transcript of the podcast, for your convenience to review in detail.

The per capita consumption of "sugar" in George Washington's day was 3 lbs/person/PER YEAR... And at the time, it was granulated sugar cane that STILL had the minerals, especially Potassium and Maggie, needed to process the Glucose in their bodies...

Today, our fellow "Colonials" are subjected to a vastly greater amount of "sugar" in their DAILY diet, but it's a FAAAAAR different beast due to:

o   Refined GMO sugar beets, that are missing the minerals...

o   High Fructose Corn (GMO) Syrup that is both cheap and wickedly destructive to our livers...

o   Toxic, synthetic sugars designed to tweak our brains!...

o   Rapidly disappearing natural sources like Honey, BSM (blackstrap Molasses), etc.

The VACUOUS DEARTH of minerals in our contemporary choice of "sweeteners" should terrify us...Tragically, MOST don't know that one of the purpose of sweetners is to fortify our minerals.

We haven't a CLUE what the collective impact of this much "sweet" is on our cells and tissues. Know that it is MOST taxing, not the least of which is the "Tax on Maggie" that this level of sweetness dictates...

The posted Infographic has *SHOCK* value that may well be worth it...

PATHOGENS (UNWANTED GUESTS)

Again, there is ALWAYS the inherent tension of "Attack the Guest!" vs "Strengthen the Host!"

I could be delusional, but I want to believe that there are TWO SIDES to this dynamic. There ALWAYS is... That said, there's NO question that Mercury is a game-changer, but I would posit, especially in a Copper-dysfunctional body -- which is the SAD state of affairs in MOST of the world...

The reality of Copper dysfunction around the world is FACT. My assessment of the INTENSIFIED state of Hg due to this lack of Copper is just a theory... however...

The body is CONSTANTLY rebuilding itself...

In the course of one hour, one Billion cells bite the dust and need to be replaced... and our body (Hypothalamus...) is directing this "re-build" 24/7... And as we provide REAL food, with REAL nutrients and minerals, our body is then able to create GENUINE replacement parts...

Delete key minerals from the operation and the body is powerless - LITERALLY... It's THAT straight forward...

http://www.goodmoodfood.net.au/#!Parasites-the-hidden-menace/c1sbz/555ea80e0cf21fee13a962c7

Parasites: the hidden menace | Good Mood Food

www.goodmoodfood.net.au

A good rule of thumb taught to us recently by a gifted Doctor of Oriental Medicine:

"Strengthen the Host... do NOT attack the Guest..."

You might take a spin through this abstract and track down the full article -- it is outstanding:

http://www.ncbi.nlm.nih.gov/pubmed/21506934

We've got to STOP attacking these "Guests," and START strengthening our "Host!", especially our Host Defense System...

The three (3) Anti-Oxidant Enzymes (SOD, CAT, GSH) are enabled and enhanced by optimal levels of bioavailable Copper and Ceruloplasmin (Cp)...

And a key activator for Cp production is Retinol, which when applied to psoriasis directly can address this vexing issue...

The FLIP-side to this dynamic is to assess Iron "deficiency" status. It has LITTLE to do with Iron and MUCH to do with Ceruloplasmin (Cp) status...

And if Cp is weak, it's a safe bet that Cu,ZnSOD is weak... And if SOD is weak, it's a safe bet that there's excess, unbound Iron that's CREATING an Oxidative Storm and ALL that "Oxidative Stress!" (That we KNOW as Rust...) is RAPIDLY aging the Thymus...And ecess, unbound Iron is breeding ground for pathogens (unwated guests).

So I think that we need to understand this - that we will increase SOD1 when we increase bioavailable Copper no matter how we do it. On the flip side, we will increase Catalase. I will try to look up a few studies in the meantime and if you don't get to do this - it is OK.

I STOPPED believing in Pasteur's FLAWED and MORONIC "Germ Theory" when I learned he was deemed a FRAUD in the NYT.... (You might enjoy reading that article...)

Copper and the PROFOUND Enzyme, Ceruloplasmin (Cp) are very much the BACK BONE of our immune system. Cp is a MAJOR Anti-Oxidant, as is the Copper-dependent SOD (Superoxide Dismutase) designed to NUKE the emissions of pathogens.

(Please know, I acknowledge that pathogens exist, I'm NOT a total Luddite, but I firmly know that in a properly mineralized body, we have INNATE IMMUNITY to defend ourselves naturally...)

In addition, another KEY Anti-Oxidant is Wholefood Vit-C that was carefully studied in the 1940's where the scientists were noting its ability to KILL H.pylori... Hmmmmm...

And what's "special" about Wholefood Vit-C?!?

It has another KEY enzyme called Tyrosinase with FOUR Copper atoms at its core...

So, I'm NOT buying your theory, even though you've found articles/books to "substantiate" your belief. Ie Ascorbic Acid.

What is imperative for you, and ALL MAG-pies, to understand is that medical research is HIGHLY political, and CAREFULLY controlled. This is very evident in the hundreds of articles that I'm now reading about Iron metabolism....

I am STUNNED by the CLEAR DIVISION in the research:

o   Articles that totally IGNORE Ceruloplasmin...

o   Articles that HONOR Ceruloplasmin... And please note, Holmberg and Laurell, who discovered Cp in the early

1940's were REVERENTIAL. The fact that they didn't get a Nobel Prize for this discovery speaks volumes about the politics of Science. (This is also evident in the failure of Friedovich and McCord to ALSO NOT get Nobel recognition for discovering SOD in the late '60's...)

I applaud your passion, and conviction, but that's not enough to sway me and hopefully the masses on MAG. I will continue to rely on the science of the superiority of Cp in the body and the cell and would invite you to "let go" of Pasteur and ask yourself HOW your "Stress!" level and mineral imbalances CAUSED your body's inability to defend itself... That is a more fruitful inquiry, in my humble opinion, and aligns far more with the purpose and focus of MAG.

Chronic bacterial infections are NOT normal, NOR natural. They are a clinical sign of "Iron Stress!" which I'm reasonably confident CAUSED BOTH the H.Pylori "infection" AND the Copper dysregulation...

IRON is THE Bad Guy -- NOT the bugs and critters! So, the REAL question is, "How'd my body get soooo "Iron Stressed!"...

I'm CERTAIN it originated with the "Stress!"-induced breakdown in your Liver's ability to MAKE Cp, for lack of bioavailable Copper, Maggie and Retinol -- the BIG THREE that would bring this VITAL enzyme to a standstill...

And ALL that ^^^^ PRECEDED the emergence and impact of H.Pylori...

I strongly advise you to watch the youtube movie on Royal Raymond Rife. He proved that a specific pathogen placed in several different mediums will result in several different growths.

It's the body's environment that brings forth the 'bugs' and depending on the medium 'your body' determines what pathogens grow.

In this case, the chicken came before the eggs...

Neither Spirulina nor Chlorella are meant to be taken on a daily basis long term.The answer to this riddle is NOT in the minerals:

http://nutritiondata.self.com/facts/custom/569428/2

But in understanding what ENZYMES the minerals MUST make:

http://www.ncbi.nlm.nih.gov/pubmed/16502333

o   Mg and Fe are KEY to Catalase...
o   Cu is KEY to making Ceruloplasmin which is
       ESSENTIAL for proper and optimal management of
       Iron...

The DANGER of these herbs, etc. is putting them in bodies that are MINERALLY DEPLETED, especially LOW in Copper and Magnesium...

Therein lies the REAL issue, in my humble opinion...

Remember, minerals are the Catalytic Keys to make Enzymes work... They are JUST like your car...Let me ask you a key question:

"When was the LAST time you drove your car WITHOUT your keys?!?..."

And when a symptom or set of symptoms arise, 100% of the time it is CAUSED by "Stress!"-induced LOSS of KEY minerals that make those activated metabolic enzymes work...

Period!

Pyroluria is one of the MOST misunderstand issues on this Planet.

Iron-induced Oxidative Stress COUPLED WITH a lack of

bioavailable Copper to make and "Iron Up!" Hemoglobin are the problems... Solve the Cu<>Fe dysregulation --due to a LACK of Cp -- and the bad guys causing the SYMPTOMS of Zn and B6 LOSS go away...

Got to pull the curtain ALL THE WAY BACK and STOP believing and basing your actions on flawed or incomplete thinking from Allopathic-land...

Simply go to Mensah's website and they explain that Oxidative Stress! is the culprit for pyroluria...

The connection IS Oxidative Stress! To LOW bioavailable Copper AND excess, unmanaged Iron is OVERWHELMING in the literature...

PROCESS OF DISCOVERY

What a HTMA Can Tell You...

HTMA and Urine are both valid ways to assess mineral status. I've no experience with the latter and don't know whether the mineral ratios metrics are the same...

When working with minerals, absolute AND relative levels are KEY...

As you might expect, there are differences in mineral presence in hair vs blood vs urine. It is very rare to see mineral studies using urine. (And In my humble opinion, the ONLY reason why organized medicine despises HTMA is that it reveals TOO MUCH!)

http://biolab.co.uk/

Remember, it's NOT the lab report, but its interpretation that is key!

Difference between mag rbc and mg HTMA

A key question is, how stable is the Mg RBC test? You can't determine a person's "stress" response from just the Mg RBC without the HTMA

Some random thoughts...

o   Heavy metal poisoning puts an enormous burden on your Detox Pathways, which are energized by Mg-ATP. You cannot make Glutathione without Mg, and nothing happens until the pathway gets energized...

o   CFS/Fibromyalgia is multi-factorial, but the lack of Mg-ATP causes muscle fibers to get "grumpy,"(p*ssed off!) and the lack of Mg in the NMDA Pain Receptors (which gets replaced with Calcium...) causes them to fire "Pain," non- stop...

o   Hippocampus is the center for memory, and is highly dependent on Mg for memory (yeah, who knew?...) and is highly sensitive to Aluminum and Copper Toxicity, again, these poisons need to be   Detoxed! -- using up more Mg-ATP...

o   Not holding adjustments is a sign of notable Adrenal Fatigue. For some reason, weak Adrenals cause ligaments and tendons to go lax... My partner, Dr. Liz (a NUCCA/network chiropractor), taught me that...

o   If your Mg is down, which is almost always is with CFS/Fibro, then your Electrolytes are not properly balanced and only add to the metabolic dysfunction taking place in your body...

OK, with those thoughts as a backdrop, beyond the HTMA, here's what I'd be seeking:

o   RBC testing of Mg, Na, and K

o   "Ionized" Calcium test

o   ATP/ADP Turnover Ratio (Mg deficiency will cause this to tank!)

o   Serum Copper

o   Serum Ceruloplasmin (transport protein for Copper)

o   Plasma Zinc

o   1,25(OH)2 D3 (Active form, aka Calcitriol)

o   Free T4 vs Free T3

o   Estrogen vs Progesterone...

That combination would provide a wide spectrum of information. Truth be known, that set of blood markers is a bit redundant to the HTMA, but as a society we are "trained" to believe that blood is best...

Hope that helps and when your results are in, I'd be happy to shed additional light on the levels and what they might mean... Blood Results combined with HTMA will give you are great overview of health.

What A HTMA Can Tell You....
By Genelle Young

When I began my journey of mineral balancing, I felt the need to know the why and how behind the diagnosis. I had tried many other avenues before going down this path, and for the first time, the evidence was right there in front of me. The more I read the more I wanted to know. With the need to read it over and over again, for it to register I put this together....

It may not be 100% correct but from my research, is was what I would refer to to see the progress my family was having. It opened my eyes to a whole new exciting world. For the first time in my 37 years the proof was in the pudding.

Morley will tell you aim of the game is to be kissing that red line.

Hair Tissue Mineral Analysis has been openly available for about the past 40 years or so. It is widely used in biological monitoring, of animal species throughout the world and is being used more and more, for human metabolic assessment as well. When understood properly, it offers great potential to improve human and animal health at the deepest levels. It can also be used preventively, and for prediction of illness.

A HTMA will supply you with reliable data on more than 35 nutrient and toxic Minerals, and over 25 important Mineral ratios. With standard blood and urine tests, valuable health information is often not revealed. Nutrient Mineral imbalances or toxic Mineral excesses that may be affecting your health, will be discovered.

Minerals are the basic 'spark plugs' of life.

Minerals are essential for growth, healing, vitality and well being. Structural support in bones and teeth, need Minerals, they also are responsible for maintaining the body's PH and water balance, nerve activity, muscle contractions, energy production and enzyme reactions.

Modern farming techniques, fertilizers and depleted soils reduce the Mineral content of foods, stripping your bodies of essential Minerals as does, environmental pollutants, chemical food additives and stressful lifestyles. All having a detrimental effect on our Mineral balance and nutritional state.

Cardiovascular disease, high cholesterol, high blood pressure, migraines, learning difficulties and hyperactivity in children, are just a few of many health conditions that are aggravated by Mineral imbalances and toxic metal excesses.

Consequently, we need to test and monitor our nutritional status more than ever.

Balancing Minerals is a journey, best traveled with an intuitive translator. A HTMA is not a form of testing we would suggest to self diagnose, or interpret. Please read the following content to give you a better understanding of the process, not to determine your status personally.

I like to focus on the first four Minerals on the grid, Ca,Mg, Na, K , as things fall into place when they are in balance. The ratios help to better understand the weakness we need to support to bring everything together.

This is not a short journey and may take a year or more to balance, but results may be seen within 3 months. Remember it took years to reach your current status.

Ratios are more important than just levels. Ratios give us the bigger picture and are indicative of disease trends. Ratios are often predictive of future metabolic dysfunction. Ratios are a great tool for charting progress as whole picture, not isolating one ratio. There are five ratios we focus on:

Calcium/Magnesium (Ca/Mg) Ratio (Blood Sugar - Cardiovascular Health)

This is often referred to as the blood-sugar ratio and is an indicator of insulin status. Calcium is needed for the pancreas to release insulin. Magnesium inhibits secretion of insulin, so it is necessary to keep calcium and Magnesium in harmony.

Ideal ratio is 7.00, however 3.4 - 9.9 is good.

Below, 3.3 is indicating you are heading to Hypoglycemia, it would indicate Magnesium loss, with possible blood sugar issues, and perhaps a hidden Na/K inversion. With 2.5 - 3.3 meaning diabetic symptoms. Any lower than 2.5 would suggest, onset of symptoms such as mental and emotional disturbances.

Above, 110 again indicates you are heading to Hypoglycemia with, tendency to insulin resistance, relative Magnesium Deficiency and possible overeating carbs. 13-18 showing diabetic symptoms, lifestyle changes needed. Any higher than 18 would suggest, onset of symptoms such as mental and emotional disturbances. High Calcium will lower cell permeability, creating a "Calcium Shell"

Magnesium or Calcium loss will raise levels temporarily, many factors can make this happen, such as Cortisone therapy lower calcium levels and will also impact Sodium and Potassium levels by raising them. Calcium can become displaced by Lead and Cadmium toxicity. I don't like to focus on the area of toxicity and prefer to balance and let the body do its job, naturally.

Sodium/Potassium (Na/K) Ratio *(Overall Vitality)*

This is a crucial ratio and often referred to as the life/death ratio, because of its importance.

The electrical potential of the cell is regulated by Sodium and Potassium, and is related to the Sodium pump mechanism, both regulating Potassium and Sodium within our body.

The ratio is an indicator of the intimate relations of the Kidneys, Liver and the Adrenal Glands functions. An imbalance of this ratio is closely associated with the Heart, Kidneys, Liver and Immune Deficiency Diseases.

This ratio gives us an indication of the Adrenal Gland function, and the balance of Cortisone and Aldosterone.

2.4 is the ideal ratio, 2.9 - 3.9 is good.

4.0 - 12 is moderate, with above 12 being extreme. High ratio would indicate, alarm reaction, acute stress, inflammation, and anger.

2.0 - 2.3 is moderately low, with 1.0 - 1.9 being serve. Below 1.00 would suggest delusional, out of touch, decreased awareness of signs and symptoms, feeling like "you are beating your head against a wall".

Na is a rough indicator of Mineralocorticoid effect (Aldosterone), pro inflammatory) K is a rough indication, of glucocorticoid effect (Cortisol), anti-inflammatory)

Na ideal is 24 - 75 alarm - 75 resist - 10 exhaust
K ideal is 10 - 5 alarm - 30 resist - 30 exhaust
ratio ideal 2.4 - 15 alarm - 2.5 resist - 0.33 exhaust

Na/K is showing signs of going into resistance stage of stress, hence the Sodium up and Potassium has come down, means it is gearing up to turn to resistance stage then exhaustion stage.

Sometimes on retesting this ratio can show worse than before, as other Minerals work so closely in relation to these two. Change in Copper status, will change this ratio as will Increase in Magnesium.

Remember Potassium in needed for your bodies to process sugar, so until you are healed, avoid sugars.

Calcium/Potassium (Ca/K) Ratio *(Thyroid)*

The Thyroid ratio because Calcium and Potassium regulate the Thyroid. Often blood tests will indicate normal ranges, whereas the HTMA will foresee the issue. Often there will be symptoms of hypothyroidism, whereas the hair test will indicate hyperactivity thyroid ratio. This is where the whole picture needs to be taken into account.

4.2 is the ideal range, 3.0 - 8.00 is a good range, with 8.1-50 being moderately Hypo, and above 50 indicating extreme Hypo.

1.0 - 2.9 would indicate moderate Hyper, and below 1.00 extreme Hyper.

Low Ca (<30) would suggest hypersensitivity, hyperkinetic, anxiety, nervousness, muscle cramps, increased permeability,unprotected psychologically, tendency to Ca deficiency.

Low K (<4) would suggest body exhaustion, but mind keeps pushing, sense of "running on fumes" and Cu toxicity regardless of Cu level and if Ca is above 50.

Thyroid proceeds Adrenals. You will not balance Thyroid until Adrenals are supported.

Sodium/Magnesium (Na/Mg) *(Adrenal)*

This ratio is referred to as the Adrenal ratio, because our Sodium levels are directly associated with the function of our Adrenals. Aldosterone, a Mineral corticoid Adrenal hormone, which regulates retention of Sodium in the body. Corticoid is any of a group of more than 40 organic compounds belonging to the steroid family and present in the cortex of the Adrenal Glands. Higher levels of Sodium would indicate, higher levels of Aldosterone.

The Adrenal ratio also measures energy output, as the Adrenals are the major Gland of the rate of metabolism.

As with the Thyroid, often blood tests will not detect an issue with the Adrenal Gland, whereas the HTMA will show the imbalance.

4.00 is the ideal ratio, with 3 - 6 being good. 6.1 - 20 would suggest moderate elevation, with tendency towards inflammation. 20+ is severe elevation, resulting in inflammation and Adrenal imbalance. Asthma, allergies, Kidney and Liver issues can be related to high ratio, that being said, high is preferred to low.

1 - 2.9 would indicate mild Adrenal fatigue, with possible digestive issues, Kidney and Liver dysfunction, allergies, arthritis, Adrenal exhaustion, deficiency of hydrochloric acid. Below 1 can indicate a tendency towards heart attacks, cancer, as well as the above symptoms. It is the state of extreme Adrenal Fatigue/ suppression.

However in saying that there have been people with a ratio below one, that were functioning well.

Sodium levels can be elevated by excess levels of several Minerals including Mercury, Iron, Copper, Cadmium, nickel. These levels will be taken into consideration when reading your HTMA.

Zinc/Copper (Zn/Cu) *(Female Hormones)*

This ratio is an effective measure of zinc and Copper readings. Elevated levels are often associated with skin problems such as, acne, psoriasis, slow healing, and eczemas. Also, emotions instability, "spaciness", PMS. Reproductive problems, menstrual issues, depression and fatigue, schizophrenia.

8.00 is the ideal ratio, with 6.5 - 10.00 being a good range. 10.1 15 is moderately high, with 15+ being extremely high. High ratios can be deceiving because of hidden Cu. With hidden Cu, the symptoms of low Zn/Cu will be present.

3.0 - 6.4 is moderately low, with below 3 being extremely low. Fast Oxidizers usually have a true low Cu and Zn. Slow Oxidizers with a low Cu usually have low bio-available Copper and excess, unbound Copper which is quiet toxic to the body.

Calcium/Phosphorus (Ca/P) (ANS State - Protein Usage)

This ratio will indicate your body's ability to break down and use Proteins.

Phosphorus levels indicates Protein usage, protein reserves and tissue breakdown. When P is low or high the following questions need to be asked, is the client eating enough Protein, from good sources, and is digestion of proteins the issue, perhaps needing HCL??

Low P is worse the high, with impaired protein synthesis being worse with low Zinc.

Ideal range is 2.63, with 2.3 - 2.8 being in the good range. 2.9 - 8.00 is moderately high with 8 and above being extremely high, Anabolic processes.

1.5 - 2.3 is moderately low, and below 1.5 being extremely, Catabolic processes.

CURRENT IDEAL HAIR MINERAL VALUES
(hair must not be washed at the laboratory for accurate readings)

MacroMinerals:

Calcium = 40 mg%
Magnesium = 6 mg
Sodium = 25 mg%
Potassium = 10 mg%
Phosphorus = 16-17 mg
Sulfur = 4500 mg%

NOTES: Sulfur usually is a little higher in fast oxidizers, up to about 5000 mg%.

Trace Minerals:

Zinc = 15 mg%,
Iron = 2 mg%,
Copper = 2.5 mg%,

 = 0.03-0.04 mg%,
Chromium = 0.06 mg%,
Selenium = 0.12 mg%,
Cobalt = 0.002 mg%,
Lithium = 0.002,
Molybdenum = 0.002,
Boron = 0.05-0.08 mg%,
Rubidium = 0.06,
Germanium = 0.003,
Iodine = 0.1 mg%,
Vanadium = 0.004 mg%,
Zirconium = 0.005 mg%
Ideal Levels Of The Toxic Minerals:

Most important toxic metals:

Lead = 0.06-0.09 mg%,
Mercury = 0.03-0.04 mg%,
Cadmium = 0.005-0.007 mg%,
Arsenic = 0.005-0.008,
Aluminum = 0.65-1.0 mg%,
Nickel = 0.02-0.04 mg%

Other toxic metals (that are much less well researched):

Uranium = 0.002-0.004 mg%,
Strontium = .008-0.01 mg%,
Antimony = 0.005-0.01 mg%,
Barium = 0.03-0.05 mg%,
Beryllium = 0.001-0.002 mg%,
Bismuth = 0.05-0.1 mg%,
Silver = 0.08-0.1 mg%,
Tin = 0.02-0.04 mg%,
Titanium = 0.05-0.07 mg%,
Platinum = 0.008-0.01 mg%,
Thallium = 0.004-0.006 mg%,
Thorium = 0.004-0.006 mg%.

Raising Minerals by lowering other Minerals

To raise Mineral:	Lower:
Calcium	Potassium
Magnesium	Sodium
Sodium	Magnesium / Zinc
Potassium	Calcium / Copper
Zinc	Potassium (if Na/K is low)
	Sodium (if Na/K is high)
Chromium	Iron / Copper / Manganese
Manganese	Iron / Copper / Calcium

Iron	Manganese / Zinc
Copper	Manganese / Zinc

The added wickedness to Copper is that ONLY "Fast" Oxidizers (20% of the population) can take Copper supplements, and the ONLY way to assess your Oxidizer pattern is through an HTMA. The notable distinction is that the Fast Oxidizer has an ability to metabolize Copper "directly", while Slow oxidizers has an equal need for bio-available Copper, but it needs to be provided "indirectly" via Wholefood Vitamin C Complex, NOT Ascorbic Acid, NOR Copper supplements, as they will only "slow" the "Slow" Oxidizer even more.

The definition of a **Fast Oxidizer** is someone with a Calcium/Potassium ratio less that 4:1 and Sodium/Magnesium ratio higher than 4.17:1. A Fast Oxidizer releases energy too fast. A Fast Oxidizer has a tendency to burn through Slow minerals like (Ca and Mg), and retain Fast minerals like (Na and K)

The definition of a **Slow Oxidizer** is someone with Calcium/Potassium ratio greater than 4:1 and Sodium/Magnesium ratio less than 4.17:1. A Slow Oxidizer releases energy too slowly. A Slow Oxidizer has a tendency to burn through Fast Minerals (Na and K), and retain Slow minerals like (Ca and Mg).

Rarely there is a **Mixed Oxidizer** that will have a Calcium/Potassium ratio greater than 4:1 and Sodium/Magnesium ratio greater then 4.17:1 or Calcium/Potassium ratio less than 4:1 and Sodium/Magnesium ratio less than 4.17:1. A mixed oxidizer has an erratic metabolism, meaning sometimes too fast, and sometimes too slow.

The **Balanced Oxidizer** is where we want to be, when the main four, Calcium, Magnesium, Sodium and Potassium are in perfect harmony. Your body is provided with perfect constant useable energy. This is bliss, happy, content, open and uncomplicated. The Balanced Oxidizer possess an inner calm and balance.

Oxidizers Patterns: Fast vs Slow

Unfortunately, Copper is NOT a straight forward shot... No, it is NOT advised to take Copper supplements unless you are a Fast Oxidizer... and the only way to know that is to complete an HTMA and learn how you relate to the Electrolytes: Calcium, Magnesium, Sodium, & Potassium...

80% of folks are Slow Oxidizers and cannot tolerate Copper straight up... 20% are Fast Oxidizers and can do so... The best & safest way to restore Copper status is wholefood Vit-C Complex -- NOT Ascorbic Acid...

Believe it or not, Fast's oxidize the Slow minerals: Calcium & Mg... and hold onto the Fast minerals: Sodium & Potassium...

And Slows do just the OPPOSITE...

No, I do NOT know why some do it this way and some the other... It is the $64 million question in the world of minerals...

The added wickedness to Copper is that ONLY "Fast" Oxidizers (20% of the population) can take Copper supplements... And the ONLY way to assess your Oxidizer pattern is through an HTMA...

I am not sold on the parameters of the "Slow vs Fast" diet as it is based on a SUBJECTIVE questionnaire, and NOT purely objective science as you might have thought...

Let's Do An HTMA with Morley Robbins

o   Hair Tissue Mineral Analysis

        http://gotmag.org/work-with-us/

o   Mg RBC (optimal is 6.0-7.0)

        http://requestatest.com/magnesium-rbc-testing

o   Signs of Magnesium Deficiencies

        http://gotmag.org/magnesium-deficiency-101/

o   How to Restore Mg:

        http://gotmag.org/how-to-restore- magnesium/

Upon ordering you will receive an email from Morley and then via snail mail which will contain the necessary scale to weigh your hair sample. Please keep these scales as that will expedite future HTMA's. On the envelope it will say Shampoo and this is asking for the brand, as certain brands have high levels of certain Minerals.

Morley M. Robbins
Nexus Whole Health
1003 E. Morris Ave.
Hammond, LA 70403 USA
Email: morley@gotmag.org
(Cell: 847.922.8061)
(Skype: morleyrobbins5)

Current turnaround time is approximately 1 month.

You will receive a customized Excel file with your ratios, graphs and over-view to discuss with Morley at your 1 hour consultation.

SAMPLE LETTER:
Dear Global Clients and MAG-pies!,

We're delighted that you've made the decision to assess your Mineral status through a Hair Tissue Mineral Analysis (HTMA). We're confident that you will find this testing procedure to be far more revealing about your body's state of metabolic balance, and the complete opposite of what you may have learned about it from prior conversations with friends, family, your doctor, or what may be posted about this process on the Internet.

Amount of Hair Required: 1 FULL Tbsp of hair (just enough to tip the cardboard Scale) in 1" - 1.5" lengths. Please **submit** from **4 spots** on your head, and please **discard** the rest of the hair. Experience has taught us that the best locations are above the ears (Temporal Lobe) and bottom of scull in the back (Occipital Lobe) -- both left and right sides.

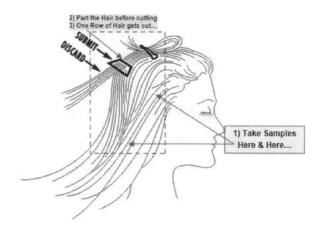

The hair needs to be washed within 24 hours and <u>dry</u> before sampling.

Place the hair sample in the small envelope with account # 6898, seal it, and then fill in your name and shampoo. Then, please complete the sections on the Blue Intake Form with RED *'s: Patient Demographic Info, Type of Shampoo, and Predominant Symptoms, *date it*, and then mail both to TEI Labs. Finally, please complete the Green Intake Form online, save it, and email it to the address noted below.

<u>BLUE INTAKE FORM and Hair</u>: <u>GREEN INTAKE FORM</u> :

Morley M. Robbins Morley M. Robbins

Nexus Whole Health   **Email:** <u>morley@gotmag.org</u>

1003 E. Morris Ave.   **(Cell: 847.922.8061)**

Hammond, LA 70403 USA **(Skype**: morleyrobbins5)

Should you be more visually inclined, please review the video link below.

<u>http://www.youtube.com/watch?v=ze8uJO-Hs_Y</u>

Please call or email me to clarify any questions that you might have about completing this sampling process.

<u>morley@gotmag.org</u>

Cheers! **Morley Robbins, *aka "Magnesium Man!"***

You can purchase a follow up consult here:

http://gotmag.org/work-with-us/

Just select the "Health Recovery Coach" option...

Turn-around time is one week to 10 days...

Metabolically active sources for HTMA:

o   Scalp Hair
o   Finger nails
o   Toe nails

Acceptable, but NOT nearly as active sources (they don't grow as much...)

o   Pubic hair
o   Armpit/Chest/Arm hair

And yes, Pubic hair skews the Phosphorus levels, but other minerals are very representative...

Assessing Your Mineral Status Via Bloods Tests

In a perfect world, I'd love to see:

http://requestatest.com/mag-zinc-copper-panel-testing?hc_location=ufi

o   Mag RBC
o   Plasma Zinc
o   Serum Copper
o   Serum Ceruloplasmin
o   Serum Iron
o   Serum Ferritin
o   Serum Transferrin
o   Serum TIBC (% SAT)

o   By far, virgin scalp hair is best...Absent that, here's the peaking order:
    -     Dyed, but NOT bleached (bleach or H2O2), is next... (Ideally, wait 4-6 weeks following your last dye session)
    -     Fingernails, next...
    -     Hair, south of the Border, is next..
    -     Your pets hair...and,
    -     Your best friend's scalp hair would be **last**...

Please check with your hairdresser to see what chemicals are used. When asked, "Shampoo?" please state brand and some brands contains high minerals.

Healthy Ranges For Blood Tests

o   Mag RBC: 5.0-7.0 mg/dL MAG goal: Strive for 6.5

o   Plasma Zinc: 100-130 mcg/dL

o   Serum Copper 80-100 mcg/dL

o   Serum Ceruloplasmin: 25-40mg/dL

o   Zinc/Usable Copper ratio: 1.3 to 1.0

o   "Usable" Copper = 3x Cp level

o   Ferritin 25-50/dL
(based on leading Cardiologists, and NOT Thyroid on
Facebook Groups lost in Iron suplementation)

Stop Supplements Before Testing

o   LabCorp has no such policy...
o   Quest says to abstain several days -- I know not why?...

This Intracellular Mg test, should be MANDATORY upon ANY doctor office visit or hospital stay. If that were the case, there would be a dramatic DECLINE in these visits...(Connect the dots, folks....)

Imagine the absurdity of an ER visit and being told to come back in 5 days when your system was "clear" of minerals!!!!

Who does that make sense to?!?...

I welcome anyone providing credible reasons why abstinence makes ANY sense for essential vital mineral tests...

Product Recommendations

When we got to this stage in the book, Morley proposed that it be discarded - at least for now. His hesitation was that he didn't want people to skip to this section, overlook the importance of having context for the symptoms that they were experiencing, and essentially "self-diagnose" with limited understanding.

It is important to know your mineral status before jumping in ANY nutrient supplementation protocol. What works for one individual, may not work for you. It is NOT a "one size fits all."

This is a brief range of a few products Morley has sourced, as he feels that they are to the highest standard.

This is a GUIDE not a diagnoses. This is a mere few recommendations, which we plan to expand over the next few books. Please remember, these companies are not affiliated with Morley, and may change their formulation at any time. If you feel there is a questionable ingredient or process, please contact Morley or the company in regards to this query.

The following recommendations have been put in here, in good faith that it is used wisely, and under the guidance of a Health Care Practitioner.

I have assured Morley, that folks who purchase these books are people who have the common sense to use these recommendations with careful consideration.

May you find what you are looking for *"A votre sante!"* - All the best, Genelle.

MTHR Natures Nutrients

Apple Cider Vinegar

Serving Size: 1 Tbsp. (15 mL)
Servings Per Container: 32
Each Serving Contains
Potassium   11mg

Blackstrap Molasses

Blackstrap molasses has very low dose of potassium, as does cream of tartar. Daily intake should be around 5000mg or more depending on your health, molasses has 1464 mg per 100gm, so that's 73.2mg per teaspoon.

What Blackstrap Molasses does for us, and for our hair - One serving (two tablespoons) of blackstrap contains approximately 14 percent of our *RDI of copper, an important trace mineral whose peptides help rebuild the skin structure that supports healthy hair. Consequently, long-term consumption of blackstrap has been linked to improved hair quality, along with the potential to encourage hair regrowth.

**Safe sweetener for diabetics - Unlike refined sugar, blackstrap molasses has a moderate glycemic load of 55. This makes it a good sugar substitute for diabetics and individuals who are seeking to avoid blood sugar spikes. Moreover, one serving of blackstrap contains no fat and only 32 calories (134 kilojoules) making it suitable for a weight loss diet when used with careful food intake. **If you should be diabetic, the use of any sugar substance should be discussed with your Medical Doctor.

Laxative qualities - blackstrap is a natural stool softener that can improve the regularity and quality of your bowel movements. Rich in iron - Two tablespoons of blackstrap contain 13.2 percent of our *RDI of iron, which our bodies need to carry oxygen to our blood cells. People who are anemic will greatly benefit from consuming 1-2 tablespoons of blackstrap molasses per day. A daily intake of blackstrap molasses can be of benefit in pregnancy, but once again, this should be discussed with your doctor.

High in calcium and magnesium - Like all whole foods, blackstrap molasses contains a mineral profile that has been optimized by nature for superior absorption. For example, two tablespoons of blackstrap contains 11.7 percent of our *RDI of calcium and 7.3 percent of our *RDI of magnesium. This calcium-magnesium ratio is ideal, since our bodies need the magnesium to help absorb the calcium. Both of these minerals aid in the growth, development and maintenance of healthy bone structure.

Additional mineral content - Two tablespoons of blackstrap molasses also contains 18 percent of our *RDI of manganese (which helps produce energy from the utilization of protein and carbohydrate), 9.7 percent of our *RDI of potassium (which plays an important role in nerve transmission and muscle contraction), 5 percent of our *RDI of vitamin B6 (which aids brain and skin development) and 3.4 percent of our *RDI of selenium, an important antioxidant.

Taking blackstrap as a health supplement The best way to take blackstrap as a supplement is to mix between 1-2 tablespoons of it in a cup of boiling water and then drink it through a straw once the water has cooled. Using a straw helps the molasses bypass your teeth. Any type of sugar coating left adhering to the teeth is not good practice. It is always beneficial for the health of your teeth and gums to clean the teeth and rinse any remaining traces of the sugar substance from the mouth.

The molasses intake ideally would be on a daily basis, and for most people, the best time is first thing in the morning.

Finally, remember to purchase only blackstrap that is organic and has not been treated with sulphur.

* Recommended daily intake.

References:-

http://www.whfoods.com

http://beforeitsnews.com

Per 2 teaspoons -

Riboflavin	.01mg	Copper	.28mg
Niacin	.15mg	Maganese	.36mg
Folate	.14mg	Selenium	2.43mcg
Vit B6	.10mg		
Calcium	117.53mg		
Iron	2.39mg		
Magnesium	29.38mg		
Phosphorus	5.47mg		
Potassium	340.57mg		
Sodium	7.52mg		
Zinc	.14mg		

Borax

(MJ Hamp's take on Borax)

A pinch in a litre of water and having one sip a day will not provide much boron.

What and How Much to Use:
In some countries (e.g. Australia, NZ, USA) borax can still be found in the laundry and cleaning sections of supermarkets. There is no "food-grade" borax available or necessary. All borax is the same and "natural", and usually mined in California or Turkey, whether it has been packed in China or any other country. The label usually states that it is 99% pure (or 990g/kg borax) which is safe to use, and is the legal standard for agricultural grade borax. Up to 1% mining and refining residues are permitted.

Boric acid, if available, may be used at about ⅔ the dose of borax, it is not for public sale in Australia.

Firstly dissolve a lightly rounded teaspoonful (5-6 grams) of borax in 1 litre of good quality water. This is your concentrated solution, keep it out of reach of small children.

Standard dose = 1 teaspoon (5 ml) of concentrate. This has 25 to 30 mg of borax and provides about 3 mg of boron. Take 1 dose per day mixed with drink or food. If that feels right then take a second dose with another meal. If there is no specific health problem or for maintenance you may continue indefinitely with 1 or 2 doses daily.

If you do have a problem, such as arthritis, osteoporosis and related conditions, cramps or spasms, stiffness due to advancing

years, menopause, and also to improve low sex hormone production, increase intake to 3 or more spaced-out standard

297

doses for several months or longer until you feel that your problem has sufficiently improved. Then drop back to 1 or 2 doses per day.

For treating Candida, other fungi and mycoplasmas, or for removing fluoride from the body - using your bottle of concentrated solution:

Lower dose for low to normal weight - 100 ml 1/8 teaspoon of borax powder or 500 mg); drink spaced out during the day.

Higher dose for heavier individuals - 200 ml 1/4 teaspoon of borax powder or 1000 mg); drink spaced out during the day.

Always start with a lower dose and increase gradually to the intended maximum. Take the maximum amounts for 4 or 5 days a week as long as required, or reduce the maximum dose for one week each month to a minimum dose, or alternatively periodically alternate between a low dose and your maximum dose in a different rhythm.

For **vaginal thrush** fill a large size gelatine capsule with borax and insert it at bedtime for one to two weeks. With **toe fungus** or athlete's foot wet the feet and rub them with borax powder.

You may take borax mixed with food or in drinks. It is rather alkaline and in higher concentrations has a soapy taste. You may disguise this with lemon juice, vinegar or ascorbic acid.
In Europe borax and boric acid have been classified as reproductive poisons, and since December 2010 are no longer available to the public within the EU. Presently borax is still available in Switzerland (15), but shipment to Germany is not permitted. In Germany a small amount (20 - 50 grams) may be

ordered through a pharmacy as ant poison, it will be registered. Borax is presently still available from www.ebay.co.uk and can be shipped to other EU countries.

Boron tablets can be bought from health shops or the Internet, commonly with 3 mg of boron.

In some European countries, such as The Netherlands, these may still contain borax, but not in others, such as Germany, where boron is not allowed in ionic form as with borax or boric acid. While suitable as a general boron supplement, I do not know if or how well they work against Candida and mycoplasmas. Most scientific studies and individual experiences in regard to arthritis, osteoporosis, or sexual hormones and menopause were with borax or boric acid. It is not yet known if non-ionic boron is as effective as borax. To improve effectiveness I recommend 3 or more spaced-out boron tablets daily for an extended period combined with sufficient magnesium and a suitable antimicrobial program (16).
Possible Side-Effects

http://www.health-science-spirit.com/borax.htm

Liver

There are just 7 different types of animal Liver.... They all have Zn<> Cu <> Fe -- in strictly different ratios.

Grass fed Beef Liver is considered, by far, the safest and the most balanced.

I would put more emphasis on Cp production and less on booga-wooga excess Copper...

This is Affagato Allopathic residue in your thinking, which is where the true "detox" needs to occur.....
If you can't eat it try desiccated liver capsule (NOT de fatted):

www.perfectsupplements.com

The Health Benefits of Perfect Desiccated Liver
Nutrient Dense Source of High Quality Protein
Boost Energy
Boost the Immune System
Boost Metabolism
Improve Digestion
Maintain Healthy Cholesterol
Maintain Healthy Blood Sugar
Maintain Cardiovascular Health
Good Source of Naturally Occurring Copper, Zinc, and Chromium High Content of Cardio-Vascular Function Boosting CoQ10 Helps Repair DNA and RNA.

Nutritional Information for Perfect Desiccated Liver Non-Defatted Grass-Fed Beef Liver
70% Protein by Weight
2.8mg of Naturally Occurring Iron per 3g Serving (Highly bio-available Form of Iron)
969 IU of Naturally Occurring Vitamin A per 3g
Naturally Occurring Vitamin B12 per 3g Serving
High Content of All B Vitamins, including B12 Potent Source of Folic Acid

LIVER There's nothing like adding bio-available Copper –

properly balanced with Zinc & Iron -- to enhance the body's stores of this vital nutrient...

I once asked one of the world's authorities on Copper, Leslie M. Klevay, MD, PhD, what the BEST source of Copper/Zinc/Iron was? His response:

Grass-fed Beef Liver! (There was NO hesitation in his response...)

He did NOT say chicken livers, duck or goose... I checked the nutrient databases for these four forms and found that the BALANCE of the Zinc/Copper/Iron was decidedly different in BEEF than the fowl...

Maybe THAT'S why our Ancestors had Beef Liver 3-4X each month...

Size of your palm, once/week...

If it's cooked with lard, onions & garlic and NOT overcooked, it's a delicacy...

All too often, it's overcooked and becomes shoe leather...

Bottom's Up!

Nutritional Yeast

I've never heard that about the use of "fotification" of nutritional yeast... The Bragg family has a long standing and sterling reputation, and I'm not aware of any issues other than the urban myth-inspired fear that this product will cause a "yeast infection" which is, simply NOT true...

But if anyone can enlighten us to the contrary, please bring it on... I want to be confident that this centuries old practice still has value today. And as far as I know, it does...

Just make sure this is NOT coming by way of Newsmax, Livestrong, Life Extension, etc... I've lost faith in many of these sites... They are fulfilling someone else's agenda -- NOT perpetuating the truth, in my humble opinion.

I often recommend the Nutritional Yeast for a natural source of B's, and the activated form of B6 to enhance cellular uptake of Mg... Given that B's are water soluble, what doesn't get used, you lose...

Vitamin B6 + Mg-ATP = > P5P (Pyridoxine-5-Phosphate). I don't know where this process occurs, but we need - 25mgs of P5P for the average person/average "Stress!" level...

As for the Mg side, most manufacturers indicate the amount of both Chelated-Mg, as well as the "elemental-Mg" that is the portion of what is available for transaction. That amount should be 5mgs/lb body weight or 10mgs/kg...

Vitamins:

Amounts Per -	16g Serving	%DV
Thiamin	9.6mg	640%
Riboflavin	9.7mg	570%
Niacin	56.0 mg	280%
Vitamin B6	9.6 mg	480%
Folate	240 mcg	60%
Vitamin B1	27.8 mcg	130%
Pantothenic Acid	1.0 mg	10%

Minerals:

Amounts Per	16g Serving	%DV
Iron	0.7mg	4%

Magnesium	24.0mg	6%
Sodium	5.0mg	0%
Zinc	3.0mg	20%
Copper	0.1mg	6%
Manganese	0.1mg	6%

Read More
http://nutritiondata.self.com/facts/custom/1323565/2#ixzz3WsVpz8QP

Olive Oil

Olive Oil is your friend to elevate Cholesterol, naturally...

The connection is that:

o Low Copper >> High Cholesterol...

o Low Manganese >> Low Cholesterol...

 Olive Oil is rich in Mn...

Adrenal Support

We regularly use this form from Medi-Herb, but it is only through practitioners:

http://www.standardprocess.com/Product/MediHerb/Ashwaganda -11#.Vkq6mxuooxq

This looks to be a good alternative also:

http://organicindiausa.com/organic-india-ashwagandha/?gclid+CNmKnsyh_clCFa5AMgodahMA1W

Australia Medi- Herb Supplier -

http://www.naturopathvitamins.com.au/index.php/test-menu-shop

Improve Respiratory Strength

Anderson's Sea Minerals...

My partner, Dr. Liz, starts the nutritional response testing with a bottle of Anderson's Sea MD.... I don't think there hasn't been a client who's neurological "lock" didn't get notably STRONGER with this mineral source in their energy field....

Aussie Sea Minerals

http://www.mmsaustralia.com.au/index.php?act=viewProd&productId=29

Serving size 5 ml (1 teaspoon, start with 5 drops and build): Ocean Derived Sea Minerals.

Contains 108 minerals, some of them are:

Sodium 90mg,
Potassium 116mg,
Calcium 0.2mg,
Magnesium 422mg,
Sulphur 69mg,
Carbon 109mg...................
250 mls (50 days supply)

Cod Liver Oil

o   Rosita's Extra Virgin CLO

Nordic Naturals has TWO versions:

o   Arctic: for those seeking CLO like their great-grandparents...

o   Arctic-D: for seeking NOT to see their grand-children...

Please note, it is the ratio of Vit-A to Vit-D that makes this product appealing, as is its processing procedure.

Retinol, animal-based Vit-A, is your best bet. (It takes 12 Beta Carotene & Zinc to equal 1 Retinol)

Beef liver & Cod Liver Oil are your richest sources. Some folks prefer desiccated tablets, but I'm assuming the potency drops, in those products due to processing... Ideally, focus on foods that will deliver all the fat soluble vitamins (A, D, E, & K)

Supplement Facts			
Serving Size: 1 Teaspoon (5 ml)			
Servings Per Bottle: 48			
	Amount Per Serving	% DV¹	% DV²ˣ
Calories	45		
Calories from fat	45		
Total Fat	5.0 g	†	8%
Saturated Fat	1.0 g	†	5%
Trans Fat	0 g	†	†
Cholesterol	20 mg	†	7%
Vitamin A	425-1500 I.U.	17-60%	9-30%
Vitamin D	0-20 I.U.	0-5%	0-5%

Total Omega-3s	1050 mg	†	†
EPA (Eicosapentaenoic Acid)	350 mg	†	†
DHA (Docosahexaenoic Acid)	485 mg	†	†
Other Omega-3s	215 mg	†	†

* Percent Daily Values are based on a 2,000 calorie diet.
† Daily Value not established.
¹ Daily Value (DV) for children under 4 years of age.
² Daily Value (DV) for adults and children over 4 years of age.

I believe your ancient ancestors INVENTED Cod Liver Oil....

WHY?

Because they knew that animal-based supplements provided ALL the nutrients & cofactors AND in the correct BALANCE.

Hormone-D MUST be balanced with 10-25X MORE retinol so that the body STAYS IN BALANCE...

Health is about Homeostasis -- NOT taking one over hyped nutrient at the expense of its biological partners in the body.

If 6 pills contain 1000IU in total of Vit-D

That level of Hormone-D needs to be matched with ~10,000 IUs of Retinol (animal-based Vit-A, NOT beta carotene, by the way...).

In my humble opinion, Carlson's is NOT a properly balanced blend... it is 2X Vit-A to 1X Vit-D...

In contrast, Nordic Naturals - Arctic is 10X Vit-A to 1X Vit-D -- THAT'S the scale of contrast needed...

When there is TOO MUCH Hormone-D, Vit-A CAN NOT do its job(s)... despite its lower cost, and it's greater popularity... Our metabolism doesn't give a lick about either one...

If you don't you run the risk of intensifying your load of bio-UN-available Copper as the lack of Vit-A will prevent production of Ceruloplasmin (Cp), which is ESSENTIAL for Copper metabolism...

Epsom Salts

Epsom salt, named for a bitter saline spring at Epsom in Surrey, England, is not actually salt but a naturally occurring pure mineral compound of magnesium and Sulfate. Long known as a natural remedy for a number of ailments. Epsom Salt has numerous health benefits within the body, including regulating the activity of enzymes, reducing inflammation, helping muscle and nerve function and helping to prevent artery hardening. Sulfates help improve the absorption of nutrients, flush toxins and help ease migraine headaches.

I would also remind you that we ARE living "1984!" where Black is white & White is black...

Examples:

o   Articles "D"emonize Epsom Salts but tell how "good" Fluoride is in our water...

o   Articles "D"emonize "grass fed" butter, yet tell us the "benefits" of GMO-laden Soy & Canola oil...

o   Articles "D"emonize Vit-A as "toxic," but glorify the use of Hormone-D...

It is ALL Affagato... It's very frustrating, but that's the world we live in now... We must challenge & question EVERYTHING that's being pumped out of Main Stream Media (whether Media or Medicine)!

Is it dangerous to take 100mg of B6 daily?
That level of B6 would likely be a good max to shoot for, but I'd ease there & not jump to that level...

Gymnema Supports Sugar Cravings

http://www.mediherb.com/product_pdf/GymnemaLR.pdf

https://www.standardprocess.com/Products/MediHerb/Gymnema#.Vsdsvgccsuk

Jigsaw Magnesium -

http://www.jigsawhealth.com/

Represented by Patrick Sullivan Jr. - Founding MAG member and one of Morley's Mentors. This is the product Morley has personally used for the past four years.

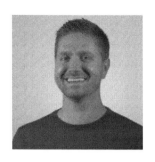

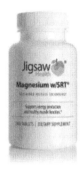

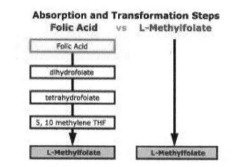

What about its Folic Acid??

It's NOT "Folic Acid..." I believe the term is "quadromethylfolate" Ask the FDA why "Folic Acid" must be used when it's not in the product...

Liver Support

Many dynamics and imbalances can affect Liver function...

o   Milk Thistle... as a herbal tonic..

Australian Stockist -

http://www.naturopathvitamins.com.au/index.php/test-menu-shop/product/34-mediherb-silymarin-milk-thistle-or-st-marys-thistle-60-tablets

o   Standard Process Livaplex… and maybe Hepatrophin PMG (it might also be advisable to do their 21-day Cleanse)

https://www.standardprocess.com/Products/Standard-Process/Hepatrophin-PMG#.Vsh59gccsul

https://www.standardprocess.com/Products/Standard-Process/Livaplex#.Vsh6p2ccsuk

o   BioRay Liver Life
http://www.bioray.com/liver-life/

Those are three very different approaches but are proven products to restore balance and function to a Liver in need.....

MolyCu

http://www.wellnessshoppingonline.com/endo-met-supplements/moly-cu-180-tabs/

ReMag

ReMag has been legendary in its ability to help folks with Mg issues. I'm not as well-versed on Re-Lyte to address Copper issues, largely because resolving Copper REQUIRES resolving Ceruloplasmin production that has been the target of dysfunction for decades & we were ALL in the "D"ark re that... You might also look into http://www.wateroz.com/ for their Cu water…

Products to help Yeast/Candida Infection

o   Probiotics are a good way to offset Yeast...
o   Wholefood Vit-C
o   Turpentine on a sugar cube (I kid you not...)
o   Bee Pollen...
o   Goat Yoghurt...
o   Goose Liver pate...
Those are all rich sources of Copper...

It needs to be ultra-distilled Turpentine: Diamand G Forest
Products in Georgia, USA is one distributor...

http://diamondgforestproducts.net/shop/32-oz-100-pure-gum-
spirits-of-turpentine/

Wholefood Vitamin C Complex

The vast majority of "Vit-C" sold and used in America/ the World
is actually Ascorbic Acid, which is only 1/6th of the Vitamin that
Albert Zvent-Gyorgi. PhD won the Nobel Prize for.

What you need is wholefood Vit-C COMPLEX"
o   Innate Response (tablets, NOT powder)
o   Grown By Nature
o   Garden of Life
o   Mega Foods
o   Standard Process (Cataplex C)
o   Pure Synergy - Pure Radiance - Organic Berries
o   Health Force Naturals - Truly Natural Vitamin C (powder)

Yes, it makes a world of difference INSIDE your body and
INSIDE your cells.....

Whole food C products - Berries ETC I'm encouraging folks to
CHECK with the manufacturers to see:

o   How much wholefood Vit-C?…

o   How much Ascorbic Acid?…

If the company cannot or will not tell you -- then that's NOT a
product you need. The ones devoted to natural wholefood Vit-C
will be delighted to tell you how much you're getting…

SELECTED BOOK REFERENCES

Among Morley's Favorites:

o   Carolyn Dean's "The Magnesium Miracle"

o   Robert G. Thompson's "The Calcium Lie I and II"

o   Andrea Rosanoff/Mildred Seelig, "The Magnesium Factor"

o   Rick Malter's, "The Strands of Health"

o   Carl C. Pfeiffer's, "Mental & Elemental Nutrients"

o   Gary Taubes', "Good Calories, Bad Calories"
    Gary Taubes', "Why We Get Fat"

o   Davis Kessler's, "The End Of Overeating"

o   Michael Pollan's, The Omnivore's Dilemma" and "Food Rules"

o   Byron Richards', "Fight For Your Health"

o   Weston A. Price's, "Nutrition and Physical Degeneration"

o   Byron J Richard's, "Mastering Leptin"

o   David L Watts, DC, PhD's "Trace Elements and Other Essential Nutrients."

o   Cate Shyamalan, MD's, "Deep Nutrition."

o   Sean Croxton's, The Dark Side Of Fat Loss"

No order of preference.

Morley's Favorite Facebook Sites:
Regarding Minerals

Magnesium Advocacy Group

https://www.facebook.com/groups/MagnesiumAdvocacy/

Copper Dysregulation and Re-balancing

https://www.facebook.com/groups/347066448791517/

Mag~nificent Mommies

https://www.facebook.com/groups/716503481736105/

Mineral Power Support

https://www.facebook.com/groups/mineralpower/

Concluding Thoughts From Morley

"The process of writing uncovers our own deepest thoughts and emotions then transforms them into a medium of teaching for others."
~ Harold Klemp ~

It is somewhat humbling to reach this point in this process... the "Conclusion" – at for Vol III!

I know for a fact, that there are other volumes of these *Musings from MAG* that are in the developmental stage, and other books planned beyond that. But, it is time for a respite from this set of reflections.

Musings is not your typical "book" and its creation is the shared collaboration of yours truly and Genelle Young, who graciously volunteered to put this set of Facebook threads together, without my knowledge, and sent it to me with an innocent question: "So, what do you think?..." The irony is that MJ Hamp, the Administrator for MAG, had undertaken that very same approach – almost two years previously. However, I was just getting my Facebook legs at the time, and was not aware of what the "potential for publishing" these daily comments and reflections were from the MAG site.

I'm walking much better, now, and I'm decidedly more awake...

It is my fervent hope that you are, as well, having gotten to this point of this document.

This book lacks the traditional trappings of most published works.It is an organic and verbatim reflection of commentary provided on the MAG website. It lacks footnotes, indexes and a story line that is typically found in the world of conventional publishing. The approach we are electing to take is one of expediency: to make these insights and observations about mineral nutrition, and its impact upon our metabolism, available to a much broader audience, given that many, many MAG-pies seem to have found them beneficial and supportive to their efforts to heal and attain mineral balance and improved well being.

But, unlike traditional books, it will have the benefit of updates and added insights as they evolve and are warranted with new information.

As I sit back and reflect on what I want you to walk away with having finished reading this document, I truly want you to do the following:

- o **Question more**....
  The REAL purpose of this book is not so much to beat my chest about what I know, but give you a very different context for the knowledge that you think you know. This book's ultimate intention is to grant you the strength of conviction to challenge what you know, and challenge those traditional sources of information. Ask more questions... do more research... exercise your critical thinking skills wherever possible – but certainly as it relates to your mineral nutrition and your health.

- o **Believe more**...
  Especially believe more in the innate capacity of your body to heal itself. Our body is designed to reach homeostasis... to get back to an even keel. Know that, and have faith in restorative powers of your body and your mind. But there is one pre-requisite: feed the body REAL food and wherever

possible, wholefood supplements. That's where the "genuine replacement parts" are for the billion cells you lose each and every hour due to the natural cycle of cell death and cell replacement. Know that your innate healer is there to serve you... it just needs to be nourished, especially with minerals. – the spark plugs of life!

o ***Share more*...**
My wildest dream is that each member of MAG will buy at least 10 copies of this book. Not because of the opportunity to make some money (although my creditors would actually like THAT for a change...), but far more importantly that this metabolic <u>truth</u> about minerals become a household phrase and way of life, that we end this tyranny of "mother may I" with mainstream medicine. I, for one, am done with that, have pledged my remaining days on this Planet to spreading that truth regularly, repeatedly, and rightfully. It's time for a much larger percentage of our world population to know these truths, as well.

o ***Express gratitude more*...**
Among the many things that I've learned over the last several years of doing wellness and HTMA consults is that when we're feeling ill, uncomfortable, or out of sync with our norm, we ALL have a tendency to find fault, express frustration and think about what we DON'T have. And how does the Universe *always* respond? By taking away EVEN MORE... So, it's time we all take stock of how to STOP that. All we need do is express heartfelt gratitude for the many, many blessings that grace our lives. And even when we're feeling our worst, there is STILL much to be thankful for. And when we engage in that regular

practice of expressing our heartfelt gratitude, despite our pains and discomfort, how does the Universe *always* respond? By giving us MORE. It never fails and that disciplined act ALSO activates the Parasympathetic Nervous System which is the side if ANS, command & control center for Rest & Recovery… the very part of our healing factors that is so often overlooked. Please, just say "Thank you!" more.

o **Gain independence more…**
At the heart of this entire effort of educating folks about minerals, and Maggie, and her Yin/Yang partner, Copper, is the expressed intention that we ALL reach a state of health independence that frees us from worry, fear, doubt, frustration and allows us to attain our TRUE purpose in this lifetime. I can assure you, we were NOT meant to suffer endlessly or stay trapped inside bodies and minds that are either NOT balanced, NOR behaving properly or fully. The more we focus on the mineral foundation that runs our body, the more we can take control of the metabolism that, in fact, runs our bodies. Again, as I've noted elsewhere in the book, there is no such thing as medical disease… there is ONLY metabolic dysfunction that is CAUSED by mineral deficiencies… That is my favorite belief and the basis of my approach to wellness coaching.

So, I will close with those thoughts.

Thank you for your time and attention. I very much appreciate the investment you have made to get to this point in the book. I also want you to know that I welcome your questions and comments about what you've read. Start a thread on MAG, drop me an email, or pick up the phone – Please know, I've NEVER met a question that I didn't enjoy. So I look forward to the feedback and the opportunity to refine this message, and address others that you, the reader, and those in you circle of family and friends, feel warrant.

70969391R00180

Made in the USA
San Bernardino, CA
09 March 2018